Macmillan / McGraw-Hill

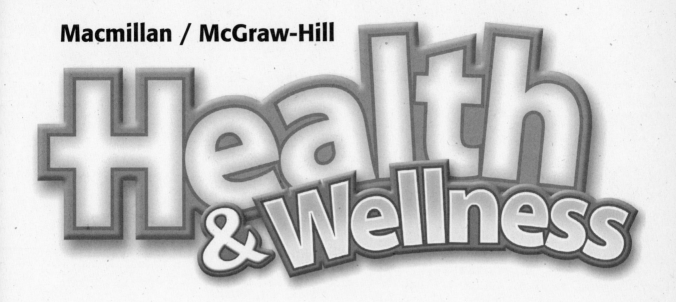

Health Masters

Grade 5

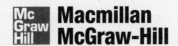

The **McGraw·Hill** Companies

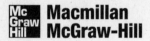
**Macmillan
McGraw-Hill**

Published by Macmillan/McGraw-Hill, of McGraw-Hill Education, a division of The McGraw-Hill Companies, Inc.,
Two Penn Plaza, New York, New York 10121.

Printed in the United States of America

1 2 3 4 5 6 7 8 9 **024** 09 08 07 06

Table of Contents

Health Behavior Contract

Name _____ Date _____

Health Goal
_____
_____

Effect on My Health
_____
_____
_____
_____
_____

My Plan
_____
_____
_____
_____
_____
_____
_____
_____
_____

My Calendar	
Monday	
Tuesday	
Wednesday	
Thursday	
Friday	
Saturday	
Sunday	

How My Plan Worked
_____
_____
_____
_____
_____
_____
_____

Name   **Date**

What Are Health and Wellness?

Directions: Write the letter of the correct answer on the line.

	Vocabulary
	A health
	B healthful behavior
	C health goal
	D life skills
	E risk behavior
	F wellness

___D___ **1.** Actions that increase and maintain your health

___C___ **2.** Something you work toward to achieve and maintain health

___F___ **3.** The highest level of health you can reach

___B___ **4.** An action that increases the level of health for you and for others

___E___ **5.** An action that can be harmful to you and others

___A___ **6.** The condition of your body and mind and the way you get along with others

Directions: Answer the questions on the lines provided.

7. How are life skills and wellness related?

By practicing life skills, you maintain and increase your health. This helps you reach wellness.

8. What are two examples of healthful behaviors?

Possible answers: washing hands often, wearing a helmet when riding a bicycle, eating healthful foods, being physically active everyday, and getting plenty of rest

9. What are two examples of risk behaviors?

Possible answers: drinking alcohol, riding double on a bike.

10. Name a health goal that you might set for yourself.

Answers will vary but should show understanding of setting goals.

What Are Health and Wellness?

Directions: Complete the lesson outline by filling in the blanks.

Health and Wellness

1. The three parts of health are:

   a. physical health _____.

   b. mental and emotional health _____.

   c. family and social health _____.

2. You have _____wellness_____ when all three parts of your health are strong.

Practice Healthful Behaviors

3. A healthful behavior is an action that _____increases_____ the level of health for you and for others.

4. Setting a _____health goal_____ of practicing healthful behaviors will help you achieve _____wellness_____.

5. A _____risk behavior_____ is an action that can be harmful to you and others.

6. You can choose _____healthful behaviors_____ to avoid _____risk_____ situations.

Top Ten Areas of Health

7. Chapter 2, Family and Social Health, describes ways to resolve _____conflict_____.

8. Chapter 4, Nutrition, identifies food choices that _____promote health_____.

9. Chapter 6, Violence and Injury Prevention, describes _____safety rules_____ for different situations.

10. Chapter 10, Environmental Health, describes how to _____conserve_____ resources.

Plan for a Healthy Life

Directions: Answer the questions on the lines provided.

1. What are health facts?

   true statements about health

2. What is reliable information?

   information that you can trust

3. How are short-term goals and long-term health goals alike?

   Both are things you work toward to improve your health.

4. How are short-term goals and long-term goals different?

   They differ in the amount of time it takes to reach the goal. Short-term

   goals can be reached in a short period of time while long-term goals

   take a longer amount of time to reach.

5. What is a health behavior contract?

   a written plan for reaching a health goal

Directions: Classify each health goal as either a *short-term goal* or a *long-term goal*.

Health Goal	Short-term Goal	Long-term Goal
6. I will eat healthful breakfasts.		x
7. I will not eat sugary snacks for two weeks.	x	
8. I will work to have healthful friendships.		x
9. I will not use tobacco.		x
10. I will help my new classmate settle in at school	x	

Plan for a Healthy Life

Directions: Complete the lesson outline by filling in the blanks.

Health Facts

1. Health facts are _____true_____ statements about health.

2. Reliable information is information you can _____trust_____.

3. Three questions you might ask to help you decide if information is reliable include:

   a. What is the source of the health facts?

   b. Is the source qualified?

   c. Are the health facts based on current scientific knowledge?

Set Health Goals

4. A health goal is something you work toward to _____achieve and maintain_____ your health.

5. Short-term goals can be part of _____long-term goals_____.

Health Behavior Contract

6. A health behavior contract is a written plan for reaching a _____health goal_____.

7. The four steps to follow when making a health behavior contract are:

   a. Write the health goal you want to set.

   b. Explain how your goal might affect your health.

   c. Describe a plan you will follow to reach your goal. Keep track of your progress.

   d. Evaluate how your plan worked.

Making a Health Behavior Contract

A Health Behavior Contract is a written plan for reaching health goals. There are four steps to follow when making and carrying out a Health Behavior Contract.

Directions: Use the chart to answer the questions.

> 1. Identify the health goal you want to set.

> 2. Tell how the goal will affect your health.

> 3. Describe a plan you will follow. Keep track of your progress.

> 4. Evaluate how your plan worked.

1. What type of information should you include in the plan you make in Step 3?
   The actions you will take to reach your goal; how you will
   monitor your progress.

2. At what point should you share your plan with your parent or guardian?
   Once the plan has been described but before beginning it.

3. Suppose your evaluation in Step 4 shows that your plan did not work. What should you do?
   Use the experience to write a new Health Behavior Contract that is
   more likely to be successful.

Your Personality and Character

Directions: Fill in each blank with the term that matches the description.

1. To treat someone with dignity and consideration is to ____respect____ him or her.

2. To have ____self-esteem____ is to have a feeling of pride in yourself.

3. Your ____personality____ is the blend of all your traits, talents, and actions.

4. A ____responsible____ person can be trusted to do what he or she says.

5. When you have ____good character____, you behave in a way that shows respect for yourself and others.

6. To have ____self-respect____ is to think highly about yourself.

7. Your ____self-concept____ is the feelings that you have about yourself.

Vocabulary

good character

personality

respect

responsible

self-concept

self-esteem

self-respect

Directions: Answer the questions on the lines provided.

8. What six traits make up good character?
trustworthiness, respect, responsibility, fairness, caring, citizenship

9. How are good character and self-concept related?
Possible answer: Developing good character keeps your
self-concept healthy.

10. How are self-concept and self-esteem related?
Possible answer: A healthy self-concept boosts your self-esteem.

Your Personality and Character

Directions: Complete the lesson outline by filling in the blanks.

Your Personality

1. Your traits, talents, and actions are part of
   your ___personality___.

2. A ___trait___ is something specific about the
   way a person acts or looks.

3. Being ___responsible___ means that you do what
   you say you will do.

Good Character

4. If you have good character, your personality includes these
   six traits:

   a. ___trustworthiness___.

   b. ___respect___.

   c. ___responsibility___.

   d. ___fairness___.

   e. ___caring___.

   f. ___citizenship___.

Self-Concept

5. Everyone has both ___strengths___ and
   ___weaknesses___.

6. Three actions you can take to keep a healthy self-concept
   are:

   a. ___improve areas where you feel weak___.

   b. ___build on your strengths___.

   c. ___develop good character___.

Your Emotions

Directions: Use the clues listed below to complete the crossword puzzle.

Across

4. A feeling inside you
5. Discomfort that results from a loss
6. A feeling of not being comfortable around other people

Down

1. A feeling of sadness and gloom
2. The state of being restless and not knowing what to do
3. A strong feeling of being irritated or annoyed

Vocabulary

anger
boredom
depression
emotion
grief
shyness

Directions: Answer the question on the lines provided.

7. What are three actions you can take to fight boredom?

Possible answers: join a club or sports group; take a class; try a new hobby

Your Emotions

Directions: Complete the lesson outline by filling in the blanks.

Feelings and Emotions

1. Understanding what you feel can help keep your
   mental and emotional health strong.

2. Three strong emotions are _anger_,
   grief, and _shyness_.

Managing Emotions

3. Three questions you can use to manage your emotions are:
   a. _What am I feeling?_
   b. _Why do I feel this way?_
   c. _How can I express what I feel in a healthful way?_

4. If you do not express anger, your _heart rate_
   and _blood pressure_ can increase.

5. Actions you can take to manage your anger in healthful
   ways include:
   a. _leave the situation and cool off_.
   b. _count to ten_.
   c. _tell the person how you feel_.
   d. _be physically active_.
   e. _ask an adult for help_.

A Healthy Mind

6. Fighting boredom helps keep your _mind_ sharp.
7. You can fight boredom by trying _new things_.

Taking Charge of Your Health

Directions: Write the letter of the correct answer on the line.

_B_ 1. A person who is the same age as you

_C_ 2. The influence people your age have on you

_E_ 3. Skills that help you to resist pressure to make a wrong decision

_D_ 4. Influence from people your age to make responsible decisions

_A_ 5. Influence from people your age to make wrong decisions

Directions: Answer the questions on the lines provided.

6. Name three influences that help you make responsible decisions.

   Possible answers: health knowledge, family, friends

7. How are positive peer pressure and negative peer pressure alike? How do they differ?

   Both refer to the influence people your age have on you. Positive peer pressure influences you to make responsible decisions, while negative peer pressure influences you to make wrong decisions.

8. Give an example of positive peer pressure.

   Answers will vary.

9. Give an example of negative peer pressure.

   Answers will vary.

10. How can resistance skills help you handle negative peer pressure?

    They give you a way to resist pressure to make a wrong decision.

Taking Charge of Your Health

Directions: Complete the lesson outline by filling in the blanks.

Making Responsible Decisions

1. If a decision is responsible, you can answer "yes" to all these questions:
   a. Is it healthful?
   b. Is it safe?
   c. Does it follow rules and laws?
   d. Does it show respect for myself and others?
   e. Does it follow family guidelines?
   f. Does it show good character?

Influences on Your Health

2. Factors that may influence your behaviors and decisions include:
   a. your personal preferences.
   b. other people.
   c. things you see and hear.

3. A classmate suggesting that you join a study group is an example of positive peer pressure.

4. A classmate urging you to smoke a cigarette is an example of negative peer pressure.

Practice Resistance Skills

5. Resistance skills help you resist pressure to make a wrong decision.

6. When using resistance skills, you should match your behavior to your words.

Managing Stress

Directions: Write the letter of the correct answer on the line.

_D_ **1.** The response to any demand on your mind or body

_E_ **2.** Anything that causes stress

_C_ **3.** Stress caused by positive events

_B_ **4.** Stress caused by negative events

_A_ **5.** A person's way of thinking and seeing things.

Vocabulary
A attitude
B distress
C eustress
D stress
E stressor

Directions: Answer the questions on the lines provided.

6. How are stressors and stress related?

Stressors cause stress.

7. How are eustress and distress similar? How are they different?

Possible answer: Eustress and distress are both types of stress, so they both have an effect on your mind and body. Eustress is a reaction to a positive stressor, while distress is a reaction to a negative stressor.

8. Give an example of something that might cause eustress.

Answers will vary.

9. Give an example of something that might cause distress.

Answers will vary.

10. Suppose you learn that you have a test today that you haven't prepared for. Describe how your body might react to this stressor.

Possible answers: I would feel worried; I would be upset; my stomach might hurt.

Name	Date

Managing Stress

Directions: Complete the lesson outline by filling in the blanks.

Everyday Stress

1. It is _____normal_____ to feel stress from time to time.

2. Stress caused by positive events is called _____eustress_____.

3. Stress caused by negative events is called _____distress_____.

4. Distress that is severe or that occurs often can _____harm your health_____.

Manage Stress

5. You can use stress management skills to _____reduce the effects of body changes_____ caused by stress.

6. Four steps to help you manage stress are:

   a. _____Identify the signs of stress._____

   b. _____Identify the cause of stress._____

   c. _____Do something about the cause of stress._____

   d. _____Take action to reduce the harmful effects of stress._____

7. Name three stress management skills.
   Possible answers: Any three: planning your time well, getting plenty of physical activity, eating healthful foods, getting plenty of sleep, avoiding food and drinks that contain caffeine, talking to your parents, guardian, or other responsible adult, trying a breathing exercise.

Coping Strategies

8. Your _____attitude_____ is your way of thinking and seeing things.

9. Your _____support network_____ is a group of people who can help you through tough times.

Make Responsible Decisions

Directions: Prepare for your role-play by completing this sheet. With your group, think of a situation in which you might have to make a tough decision. Then list three choices. Evaluate each choice and identify your decision. The four steps are listed to the right as a reminder.

1. Identify your choices.

2. Evaluate each choice. Use the *Guidelines for Making Responsible Decisions*™.

3. Identify the responsible decision.

4. Evaluate your decision.

1. Describe the situation.

   _____

2. List three choices.

   a. _____

   b. _____

   c. _____

3. For each choice ask:

	Choice 1	Choice 2	Choice 3
Is it healthful?			
Is it safe?			
Does it follow rules and laws?			
Does it show respect for myself and others?			
Does it follow family guidelines?			
Does it show good character?			

4. Identify your decision. Describe it and explain why you chose it.

   _____

   _____

   _____

   _____

   _____

Your Social Health

Directions: Write the letter of the correct answer on the line.

B	**1.**	The high regard that two people have for each other
D	**2.**	A person whose behavior other people copy
C	**3.**	A connection you have with another person
A	**4.**	A person who helps keep others healthy

Vocabulary

A health advocate

B mutual respect

C relationship

D role model

Directions: Describe each relationship listed below on the lines provided. Include the behaviors displayed by the people in each relationship.

5. Family
   a. shares loving relationships
   b. gives support
   c. meets needs such as food, shelter, and clothing
   d. helps you develop in healthful ways

6. Friends
   a. help you learn who you are apart from your family
   b. support each other
   c. influence each other in positive ways

7. Limited relationship
   a. rely on another for a special service

Directions: Answer the question on the lines provided.

8. Think of a person who is or could be a positive role model for you. Describe what you admire about this person and what behaviors you would like to copy.

   Answers should reflect a person with healthful behaviors.

Your Social Health

Directions: Complete the lesson outline by filling in the blanks.

Kinds of Relationships

1. The three kinds of relationships include
   a. ___family___,
   b. ___friends___, and
   c. ___others, or limited relationships___.

Begin with Respect

2. People are different in many ways. Four of them are:
   a. ___They speak different languages___.
   b. ___They come from different parts of the world___.
   c. ___They have different beliefs and interests___.
   d. ___They may have special needs___.

3. Make people who are different from you feel welcome by
   a. ___starting a conversation with them___;
   b. ___walking home with them after school___;
   c. ___introducing them to other friends___; and
   d. ___asking them to join you in an activity after school___.

4. To earn the respect of others, you should treat them
   with ___respect___.

5. When there is ___mutual respect___, two people see
   each other as equally important.

Be a Health Advocate

6. The four steps in becoming a health advocate are:
   a. ___Choose a healthful action to communicate___.
   b. ___Collect information about the action___.
   c. ___Decide how to communicate this information___.
   d. ___Communicate your message to others___.

Communication in Relationships

Directions: Fill in each blank with the term that matches the description.

1. An effective way to communicate feelings
is an _____I-message_____.

2. To exchange or share ideas, information, and
feelings is to _____communicate_____.

3. The movements or gestures people make when
communicating with another person are
_____body language_____.

Vocabulary

body language

communicate

I-message

Directions: Answer the questions on the lines provided.

4. What does an I-message do?
It states the problem and tells how it affects you; it doesn't
blame others.

5. What is communicating without words?
nonverbal communication

6. What is posture?
the way you hold your body

7. What is just as important as talking when communicating?
listening

8. What are two parts of active listening?
attending and acknowledging

9. What are three tips for good listening?
Any three: make eye contact, use gestures, lean toward the speaker,
don't interrupt, repeat what was said to make sure that you
understand it

10. What is the key to managing strong emotions?
self-control

Communication in Relationships

Directions: Complete the lesson outline by filling in the blanks.

Healthful Communication

1. Healthful communication can help you develop
   strong and trusting relationships.

2. Communication can be difficult when people
   do not agree on what decision to make.
   _____ Emotions _____ can also make communication
   difficult.

3. Use _____ I-messages _____ to explain how you feel
   and avoid putting someone else down or placing blame.

Nonverbal Communication

4. You may say more through your _____ body language _____
   than through your words.

5. _____ Facial expressions _____ and _____ posture _____
   reveal a great deal about how you feel.

6. Active listening includes _____ attending _____, or
   paying attention. Active listening also includes
   _____ acknowledging _____ what you hear.

Communicating Emotions

7. You may need to learn to _____ manage _____ strong
   emotions.

8. Tips to use if you feel angry include:

   a. _____ Stop _____.

   b. _____ Take time out _____.

   c. _____ Think about the situation _____.

   d. _____ Act on your decision _____.

Name   **Date**

When Conflict Occurs

Directions: Fill in the blanks in the puzzle. Use the terms that match the descriptions. Write each letter that has a number below it on the line with the matching number at the bottom of the page. Read the decoded sentence.

Vocabulary		
conflict	mediation	peace
prejudice	stereotypes	violence

1. Overly simple opinions or attitudes about certain groups of people are

   <u>s</u> <u>t</u> <u>e</u> <u>r</u> <u>e</u> <u>o</u> <u>t</u> <u>y</u> <u>p</u> <u>e</u> <u>s</u> .
    3   1   15

2. Being free of unsettled conflict within yourself or with others is

   <u>p</u> <u>e</u> <u>a</u> <u>c</u> <u>e</u> .
   12

3. A disagreement or fight is

   <u>c</u> <u>o</u> <u>n</u> <u>f</u> <u>l</u> <u>i</u> <u>c</u> <u>t</u> .
         4   9   11

4. A type of intervention to resolve conflict is

   <u>m</u> <u>e</u> <u>d</u> <u>i</u> <u>a</u> <u>t</u> <u>i</u> <u>o</u> <u>n</u> .
        2   13   8

5. An act that harms you, others, or property is

   <u>v</u> <u>i</u> <u>o</u> <u>l</u> <u>e</u> <u>n</u> <u>c</u> <u>e</u> .
    6   5   7

6. An opinion that is formed before all the facts are known is

   <u>p</u> <u>r</u> <u>e</u> <u>j</u> <u>u</u> <u>d</u> <u>i</u> <u>c</u> <u>e</u> .
             14   10

   <u>R</u> <u>e</u> <u>s</u> <u>o</u> <u>l</u> <u>v</u> <u>e</u>   <u>c</u> <u>o</u> <u>n</u> <u>f</u> <u>l</u> <u>i</u> <u>c</u> <u>t</u>
    1   2   3   4   5   6   2   7   4   8   9   5   10   7   11

   <u>p</u> <u>e</u> <u>a</u> <u>c</u> <u>e</u> <u>f</u> <u>u</u> <u>l</u> <u>l</u> <u>y</u> !
   12   2   13   7   2   9   14   5   5   15

When Conflict Occurs

Directions: Complete the lesson outline by filling in the blanks.

How Conflict Develops

1. Two types of conflict are
   a. _____inner conflict_____, and
   b. _____interpersonal conflict_____.
2. Conflict can occur because of _____cultural differences_____
   and _____prejudice_____.
3. Stereotypes are overly simple _____opinions_____ or
   _____attitudes_____ about a group of people.

When Conflict Mounts

4. Unresolved conflict may lead to _____violence_____.
5. Remember to use _____I-messages_____ and active
   listening when expressing your _____thoughts and feelings_____.
6. List the four steps in resolving conflict.
   a. _____Stay calm_____.
   b. _____Talk about the conflict_____.
   c. _____List possible ways to settle the conflict_____.
   d. _____Agree on a responsible way to settle the conflict_____.
   You may need to ask a trusted adult for help.

When to Get Help

7. When it is hard to arrive at a solution, _____mediation_____
   may be needed.
8. If you are part of mediation, _____be respectful_____,
   _____work together_____, and be prepared to
   _____give and take_____.

Ways to Resolve Conflict

Directions: Use the chart to answer the questions.

Instead of THIS:	Try THIS:
letting a situation get too serious	using communication skills to keep the situation calm
punching someone	talking about the situation
hiding what you feel	expressing it in a healthful way
teasing people who are different from you	getting to know them so that you can understand them better

1. What kind of information does this chart provide?

   behaviors or actions that can cause conflict and the behaviors you can

   use to help prevent conflict

2. Which column shows the problem behaviors?

   the first column

3. Instead of allowing a situation to get too serious, what could you do?

   use communication skills to keep the situation calm

4. Instead of teasing people who are different from you, what could you do?

   get to know them so that you can understand them better

5. List one more problem behavior and one more tip to prevent the problem to add to this chart.

Instead of THIS:	Try THIS:
Possible answer: blaming another person for something that went wrong	Possible answer: talking with the person to find a way to correct the situation or problem

Health in the Family

Directions: Write the letter of the correct answer on the line.

E   **1.** traits you get from your birth parents

B   **2.** everything around you

C   **3.** a group of people who are related in some way

F   **4.** your way of living

A   **5.** being willing to work together

D   **6.** your usual way of doing things

Vocabulary
A   cooperative
B   environment
C   family
D   habit
E   heredity
F   lifestyle

Directions: Answer the questions on the lines provided.

7. What are four kinds of families?

The four kinds of families are a nuclear family, a single-parent family,

a blended family, and an extended family.

8. What are family guidelines?

Family guidelines are rules that guide children to act in ways that protect

their health and safety and develop good character.

9. Write a short paragraph explaining how your family influences your health.

Answers should include a discussion about the influence of family on

heredity, habits, and environment.

_____

_____

_____

_____

_____

_____

_____

_____

Health in the Family

Directions: Complete the lesson outline by filling in the blanks.

Kinds of Families

1. Kinds of Family	Description of Members
Nuclear family	a. *a husband and wife who raise one or more children*
b. *Single-parent family*	One parent who raises one or more children
c. *Blended family*	One or both parents have been married before; children from either parent
Extended family	d. *Relatives, such as grandparents, who might act as guardians*

2. Healthy family members are ____*cooperative*____, or willing to work together.

3. Family guidelines are rules set by ____*parents or guardians*____ to protect children's ____*health and safety*____ and to help them develop ____*good character*____.

Family Influences on Your Health

4. You may see your heredity in your ____*appearance*____ and your ____*talents*____. Heredity may also increase the risk of ____*some diseases*____.

5. A ____*healthful*____ family environment helps keep family members ____*healthy*____ and ____*safe*____.

6. If a child's physical needs are not met, the child may not ____*grow and develop*____ normally. If a child's emotional needs are not met, the child may not learn how to have ____*caring and respectful*____ relationships and express feelings in ____*peaceful and healthful*____ ways.

Facing Family Challenges

Directions: Fill in each blank with the term that matches the description.

Vocabulary

abuse
adoption
divorce
foster child
neglect
separation

1. A child who lives in a family without being related by birth or adoption is a(n) __foster child__.

2. To treat roughly or harshly is to __abuse__.

3. A legal end to a marriage is a(n) __divorce__.

4. Parents take a child of other parents into their family to make that child their own through __adoption__.

5. The lack of attention or care is __neglect__.

6. A(n) __separation__ occurs when a couple is still married, but the husband and wife are living apart.

Directions: Answer the questions on the lines provided.

7. How can divorce affect a child's health?

   It can make a child feel very sad even though he or she is not to blame.

8. How might parents who are separated or divorced and their children deal with the changes that result from the situation?

   Talking helps children and their parents deal with the changes.

   Children and parents can talk to counselors, religious leaders,

   doctors, and social workers.

9. Which two vocabulary terms are sometimes associated with a family member's choosing a risk behavior, such as drinking alcohol?

   abuse and neglect

10. What is the difference between a foster child and a child who is adopted?

    A foster child lives in a family without being related by birth or adoption.

    A child who is adopted becomes a permanent part of the family.

Facing Family Challenges

Directions: Complete the lesson outline by filling in the blanks.

Family Balancing Act

1. Family Members	Responsibilities
Parents, stepparents, and guardians	a. Earn an income b. Cook c. Clean d. Take care of needs of other family members
Children	a. Do chores

2. The benefits of children sharing work are:

   a. family members can spend more time together .

   b. children learn skills that they will use when they have homes of their own .

Growth and Change

3. A family may grow in size because a child is _____born_____ or _____adopted_____ into the family.

4. When a family grows, other children may feel _____happy_____ , _____sad_____ , or _____jealous_____ .

5. Sharing _____feelings_____ with a _____family member_____ can help children adjust to family growth.

6. Usually parents can _____solve problems_____ in their marriage. If they cannot, they may decide to _____separate_____ .

7. When parents can't solve their problems, they may get a _____divorce_____ , which is a _____legal end_____ to a marriage.

continued

continued

8. Yelling at or hitting family members is a kind of
_____ abuse _____. Not taking care of a child's
needs is _____ neglect _____.

9. Abuse and neglect can be caused by
_____ drug and alcohol abuse _____ or by _____ stress _____
that is not handled in healthful ways.

10. Family members can seek outside help during challenging
times from

a. _____ school counselors _____.

b. _____ clergy _____.

c. _____ doctors _____.

d. _____ social workers _____.

Family Ties

11. Family members strengthen their bonds with each other by

a. _____ making time to talk to each other _____.

b. _____ showing respect for each other _____.

c. _____ considering each other's feelings _____.

12. In healthy families, family members resolve conflicts by

a. _____ listening to what each other has to say _____.

b. _____ cooperating to work things out _____.

c. _____ apologizing for problems they may have caused _____.

d. _____ solving problems in ways that agree with family guidelines _____.

Family Chore Schedule

Directions: Use the chore schedule to answer the questions.

Family Chore Schedule				
	Mom	Dad	Jesse	Grace
Every day	Fix dinner Drive children to school	Fix breakfast Pack lunches Make bed	Do the dishes Feed the dog Make bed	Set and clear the table Walk the dog Make bed
Once a week	Clean the bathroom Do laundry	Mow the lawn Clean the kitchen	Clean my room Vacuum the house	Clean my room Water the plants

1. What jobs does Jesse do every day?
   do the dishes, feed the dog, make the bed

2. Which jobs does Grace do once a week?
   clean her room, water the plants

3. Why might some chores be done only once each week?
   Possible answers: It is unnecessary to perform some chores more
   than once each week; some require more time than is available during
   other days

4. List three advantages of making a schedule to do chores.
   Possible answers: A schedule acts as a reminder; it makes doing
   certain tasks a priority on certain days; it's a way to be sure that
   everything that needs to be done is accomplished

Among Friends

Directions: Use the clues to complete the puzzle.

Across

3. skills that help you interact with others
4. a process in which two people develop feelings of closeness for one another

Down

1. a person who likes and supports you
2. a group of people who stick together and are often unfriendly to people outside the group

Vocabulary
bonding
clique
friend
social skills

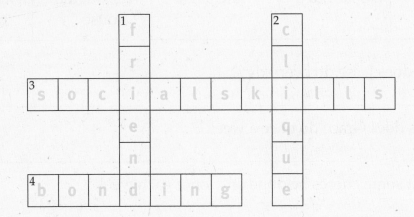

Directions: Answer the questions.

5. What are three qualities of a friend?

Accept any three of the qualities from the checklist on page A75.

6. What process allows friends to become close?

bonding

7. In what ways do members of cliques hurt themselves?

They hurt themselves because they have fewer friends and fewer opportunities to develop new social skills.

Name   Date

Among Friends

Directions: Complete the lesson outline by filling in the blanks.

Friendship and Social Skills

1. Friends can help you improve your _____ social _____ skills. These skills help you _____ interact with others _____.

Making Friendships Stronger

2. Some guidelines for friendship are:

   a. _____ Make responsible decisions with friends _____.

   b. _____ Keep confidences whenever possible _____.

   c. _____ Talk over disagreements _____.

   d. _____ Keep your promises _____.

   e. _____ Encourage each other to grow _____.

   f. _____ Allow each other time to be alone and to be with family members and other friends _____.

3. You should tell an adult if a friend's secret involves something _____ illegal _____ or that could be _____ harmful to your friend or to others _____.

Cliques Can Be Harmful

4. Members of cliques may _____ tease _____ or _____ refuse to talk to _____ people who are not in the clique.

5. People who join cliques may have _____ fewer _____ friends and less chance to learn _____ social skills _____.

6. Four ways to avoid cliques and build your social skills are:

   a. _____ Include new people in your group of friends _____.

   b. _____ Go out of your way to meet people _____.

   c. _____ Say "no" if your group of friends wants to leave others out for no good reason _____.

   d. _____ Get together with others in healthful ways _____.

Facing Challenges in Relationships

Directions: Fill in each blank with the term that matches the description.

1. A person who likes to threaten and frighten others is
   a ___bully___.

2. A place on the Internet in which people can have live discussions with one another is called
   a ___chat room___.

Vocabulary
bully
chat room

Directions: Answer the questions.

3. What is peer pressure?
   the influence of people your own age to go along with their beliefs
   and activities

4. What type of influence do you experience when a friend tries to get you to do something that you know is wrong?
   negative peer pressure

5. Write a paragraph about the dangers of chat rooms.
   Answers should include that people of all ages can use them and
   that students may not know who the people in the chat room are.

6. List two guidelines for using chat rooms.
   a. avoid them _____ or
   b. enter only those that your parents or guardian approve.

7. List three ways you can avoid being threatened by a bully.
   a. Change your routes.
   b. Change the times that you do things.
   c. Stay with groups of friends.

Facing Challenges in Relationships

Directions: Complete the lesson outline by filling in the blanks.

Peer Pressure

1. The influence that people your age have on you is
   _____peer pressure_____.

2. You can avoid bullies by _____changing your routes and times_____
   and _____staying with groups of friends_____.

3. When a friend pressures you to make a wrong decision,
   it's important to:
   a. _____match your actions to your words_____.
   b. use _____resistance skills_____ and
      _____the Guidelines for Making Responsible Decisions™_____.
   c. _____suggest another activity that you can enjoy_____.

4. Five reasons that you can give to avoid risk behaviors when
   peers pressure you include these:
   a. _____Accept any five from the list on page A81._____.
   b. _____.
   c. _____.
   d. _____.
   e. _____.

Negative Influences

5. TV and movies don't show the harm that
   _____risk behaviors_____ can cause.

6. It is best to _____avoid_____ chat rooms or use only those
   that your _____parents or guardian_____ approves.

Use Resistance Skills

Directions: Suppose a friend asks you to play a game. Your parents have said you can't play until your homework is done. Your friend suggests that you tell your parents that you have no homework. With a group of classmates, role-play how to say "no" to your friend in this situation. The role-play should show how to use resistance skills to say no. The skills are listed to the right as a reminder. Write down your answers.

Use Resistance Skills
1. Look at the person. Say "no" in a firm voice.
2. Give reasons for saying "no."
3. Match your behavior to your words.
4. Ask an adult for help if you need it.

1. What are some possible reasons you can give for saying no to your friends?

   Possible answers: "I want to follow our family guidelines";

   "I want to get my homework done so I can play later."

2. How can you make sure your body language supports what you are saying?

   Possible answers: Have good posture and stand up straight; be firm

   when you speak; make eye contact when saying "no."

3. If your friends continue to pressure you or tease you for not following along, who could you talk to about it?

   Possible answers: parent or guardian, teacher, counselor

Extend

Think about how the steps for using resistance skills might apply to the following situations. List the reasons from page A81 that would be most appropriate.

a. A friend wants you to be a lookout while he or she steals a candy bar.

   _____

   _____

b. A friend asks you to play a mean prank on a new student.

   _____

   _____

Your Body's Systems

Directions: Write the letter of the correct answer on the line.

___D___ **1.** The framework that supports the body and helps protect internal tissues

___A___ **2.** A group of organs that work together to carry out certain tasks

___B___ **3.** When body systems rely on one another to work

___C___ **4.** What helps the body move and maintain posture

Vocabulary
A body system
B interdependence
C muscular system
D skeletal system

Directions: Fill in each numbered blank in the table with the correct term.

Body System	Its Parts	Its Functions
Muscular system	Bones 5. _Muscles_	Moves the body 6. _Maintains posture_
7. _Skeletal system_	Joints Ligaments 8. _Bones_	Supports the body Moves the body 9. _Protects internal tissues_

Directions: Answer the question on the lines provided. Use complete sentences.

10. Give an example of the interdependence of body systems.

Possible answers: The skeletal system and muscular system work together and allow the body to move. The circulatory system brings air from the respiratory system and food from the digestive system to body cells.

Name _____ **Date** _____

Your Body's Systems

Directions: Complete the lesson outline by filling in the blanks.

Cells, Tissues, Organs, and Body Systems

1. The smallest living part of your body is a _____ cell _____.

2. A group of cells that work together is a _____ tissue _____.

3. A group of tissues that work together is an _____ organ _____.

4. A _____ body system _____ is a group of organs that work together to carry out certain tasks.

Bones and Muscles

5. The _____ skeletal _____ system supports the body and protects internal tissues.

6. A _____ joint _____ is where two bones meet.

7. The _____ muscular _____ system helps you move and maintain posture.

8. Your bones and muscles work together to support and _____ move _____ your body.

9. Muscles and bones connect to one another through bands of tissues called _____ tendons _____.

10. Muscles that you can control are called _____ voluntary _____ muscles.

11. You can care for your bones and muscles by

    a. selecting foods and drinks high in _____ calcium _____, such as cheese and milk.

    b. getting a lot of _____ physical _____ activity.

    c. using safety gear, such as a _____ helmet _____.

Body Systems Working Together

12. Body systems rely on one another to work properly. This is called _____ interdependence _____.

The Skeletal System

Directions: The diagram shows the bones that make up the skeletal system. Use the diagram to answer the questions.

1. Where in the body are these bones found?

   a. femur _____leg or thigh_____

   b. humerus _____arm_____

   c. vertebrae _____back or torso_____

2. Which internal organs do these bones protect?

   a. ribs _____heart, lungs_____

   b. skull _____brain, eyes_____

3. Which joints are hinge joints?

   _____elbow, knee, fingers, toes_____

4. What kind of movement do hinge joints allow?

   _____open-and-close movements that operate_____

   _____like a door hinge_____

5. What kind of movement do ball-and-socket joints allow?

   _____circular movements_____

6. What kind of movement do the joints in the skull allow?

   _____no movement_____

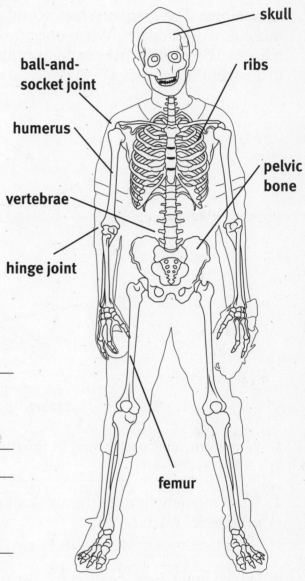

skull

ball-and-socket joint

ribs

humerus

pelvic bone

vertebrae

hinge joint

femur

How Muscles Work

Directions: The diagram shows how voluntary muscles in the arm work. These muscles work in pairs. When one muscle in a pair contracts, the other muscle relaxes. The muscle that contracts pulls a bone in one direction. Use the diagram to answer the questions.

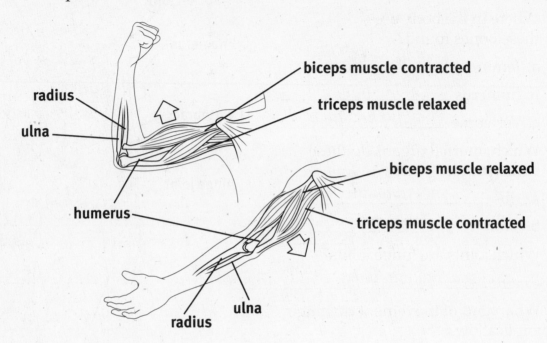

radius
ulna
biceps muscle contracted
triceps muscle relaxed
biceps muscle relaxed
humerus
triceps muscle contracted
ulna
radius

1. Which muscles are shown in the diagram?

   biceps and triceps
   _____

2. What movement does the arm make when the biceps muscle contracts?

   The arm bends at the elbow joint.
   _____

3. Which bone does the biceps muscle pull? Where is the biceps muscle in the body?

   the radius; in the upper arm
   _____

4. How does the biceps muscle change when it contracts?

   It gets shorter.
   _____

5. What movement does the arm make when the triceps muscle contracts?

   It straightens out.
   _____

6. Which bone does the triceps muscle pull?

   the ulna
   _____

Name   **Date**

Your Heart and Lungs

Directions: Write the letter of the correct answer on the line.

E   **1.** Removes oxygen from the air you breathe

D   **2.** Breathe out

F   **3.** Vessels that carry blood to the heart

A   **4.** Short tubes that carry air to your lungs

C   **5.** Takes blood and oxygen to all the body's cells

B   **6.** Waste gas made by the cells

Vocabulary
A bronchi
B carbon dioxide
C circulatory system
D exhale
E respiratory system
F veins

Directions: Use the words below to complete the chart.

alveoli	arteries	blood	bronchioles	capillaries
heart	lungs	nose	trachea	veins

Parts of the Circulatory System	Parts of the Respiratory System
7. heart	**8.** alveoli
9. arteries	**10.** bronchioles
11. blood	**12.** lungs
13. capillaries	**14.** nose
15. veins	**16.** trachea

Your Heart and Lungs

Directions: Complete the lesson outline by filling in the blanks.

Your Heart

1. The _____circulatory_____ system transports oxygen, food, and waste through the body.

2. Your heart pumps _____blood_____ to your body's cells.

3. Blood vessels that carry blood away from the heart are called _____arteries_____.

4. Blood vessels that bring blood back to the heart are called _____veins_____.

5. Tiny blood vessels are called _____capillaries_____.

6. Three ways to take care of your circulatory system are
   a. Get plenty of _____physical activity_____.
   b. Limit _____fatty foods_____.
   c. Have a plan to manage _____stress_____.

Your Lungs

7. The _____respiratory_____ system helps the body use air.

8. Air enters the body through the _____nose and mouth_____.

9. After air enters the body, it first moves to the _____trachea_____. Then it passes through tubes called _____bronchi_____ into the _____lungs_____. These tubes branch into _____bronchioles_____, which end in _____alveoli_____.

10. Capillaries carry _____oxygen_____ from the _____alveoli_____ to the body.

11. Three ways to take care of your respiratory system are
    a. get plenty of _____physical activity_____.
    b. avoid breathing _____poisonous fumes_____.
    c. avoid _____smoking_____.

The Respiratory System

Directions: The diagram shows the parts of the respiratory system. Use it to answer the questions.

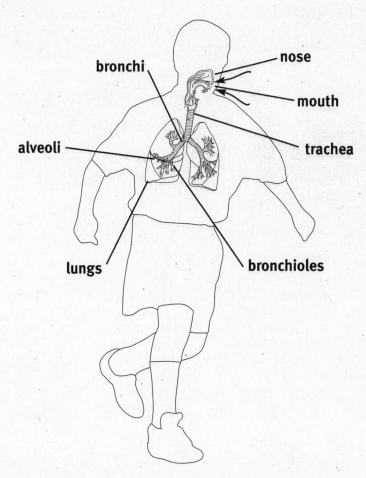

1. Through which two organs does air enter the body?
   nose and mouth

2. Through what passage does air get into your lungs?
   trachea

3. Through which organs does air leave the body?
   nose and mouth

4. Doctors use a stethoscope to listen to some body systems.
   Study the diagram. What do doctors hear when a person
   takes a deep breath and releases it?
   air moving into and out of the lungs

The Circulatory System

Directions: Look at the diagram of the circulatory system. Use the diagram to answer the questions.

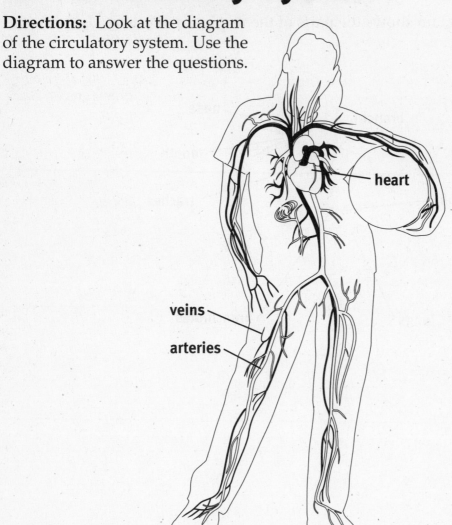

heart

veins

arteries

1. Where in the body are the veins and arteries?
   throughout the body
   _____

2. Where do the veins and the arteries start?
   the heart
   _____

3. Describe how blood moves through the body.
   Possible answer: Blood flows out of the heart through arteries to the
   body. It then flows back to the heart through veins.
   _____
   _____
   _____

More Body Systems

Directions: Use the clues to complete the puzzle.

Across

1. The _____ system controls all the functions of the body.
3. The _____ system breaks down food so that it can be used by your body.
6. The stage of life when a person's body becomes able to reproduce is called _____.
7. The _____ system is made up of glands.

Down

2. The _____ system removes liquid wastes and other materials from the blood.
4. Substances in food that your body needs for energy, to repair itself, and to grow are called _____.
5. A chronic disease in which there is too much sugar in a person's blood is called _____.

Vocabulary
diabetes
digestive
endocrine
nervous
nutrients
puberty
urinary

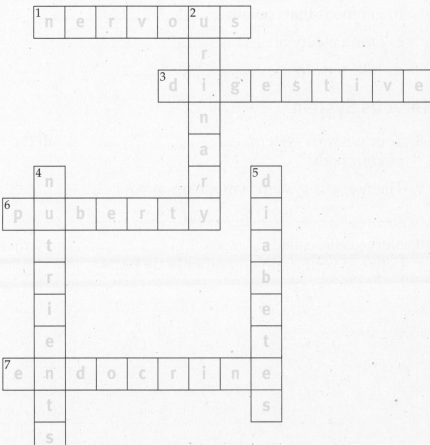

More Body Systems

Directions: Complete the lesson outline by filling in the blanks.

Digestive System

1. Food begins to break down in the _____ mouth _____.

2. The teeth chew food and mix it with _____ saliva _____.

3. The _____ tongue _____ pushes food into the esophagus.

4. In the stomach, _____ digestive juices _____ break down the food more.

5. From the stomach, food moves into the _____ small intestine _____.

6. Capillaries in the small intestine absorb _____ nutrients _____.
   The blood carries them to _____ body cells _____.

7. Four ways to take care of your digestive system are:

   a. Always _____ chew _____ your food well.

   b. Eat foods that contain _____ fiber _____.

   c. Drink plenty of _____ water _____.

   d. Take time to _____ relax _____.

Nervous System

8. Your nervous system _____ controls _____ all the functions of your body.

9. The nervous system is made up of your _____ brain _____, _____ spinal cord _____, and _____ nerves _____.

10. Nerve cells, called _____ neurons _____, carry messages between your brain and other body parts.

continued

Name   **Date**

continued

11. The brain has three main sections:

   a. The _____ cerebrum _____ controls learning, memory, and voluntary movements.

   b. The _____ cerebellum _____ makes sure your muscles work well together.

   c. The brain _____ stem _____ controls involuntary actions, such as your heartbeat.

12. The spinal cord is a thick band of _____ nerves _____ that carries messages to and from the brain.

13. A _____ reflex _____ is a quick reaction, such as when a person touches something hot. Nerves in the spinal cord respond without _____ waiting for messages from the brain _____.

14. Care for your nervous system by

   a. wearing a _____ seat belt _____ in the car and a _____ helmet _____ when playing sports.

   b. avoiding _____ drugs _____ and _____ breathing poisonous fumes _____.

Endocrine and Urinary Systems

15. Endocrine glands make _____ hormones _____ that control _____ specific body activities _____.

16. The pituitary gland makes a _____ growth _____ hormone.

17. The stage in life when a person's body becomes able to reproduce is called _____ puberty _____.

18. Your urinary system removes _____ liquid wastes _____ from the _____ blood _____.

19. The _____ kidneys _____ remove wastes and mix them with water to form _____ urine _____, which is held in the _____ bladder _____.

Digestive System

Directions: The diagram shows the parts of the digestive system. Use it to answer the questions.

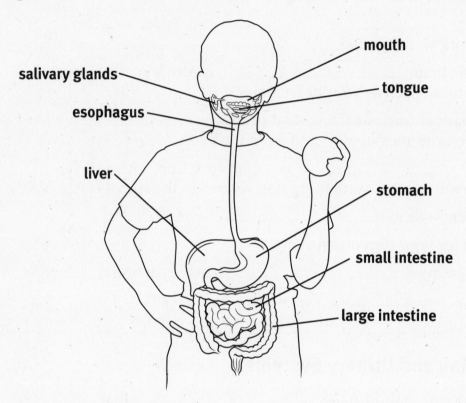

1. Where does digestion begin?

   mouth
   _____

2. After leaving the mouth, where does food move to?

   the esophagus
   _____

3. Where does food move from when entering large intestine?

   small intestine
   _____

4. What parts in the mouth aid in digestion?

   tongue and salivary glands
   _____

5. What part of the digestive system shown does food not travel to?

   liver
   _____

Name   **Date**

Nervous System

Directions: The diagram shows the parts of the nervous system. Use it to answer the questions.

1. Where in the body are the nerves?

   all over the body

2. From where do the nerves branch out?

   the spinal cord and the

   brain stem

3. How might an injury to the spinal cord affect the nerves?

   It could affect communication between

   the body and the brain.

4. What are the main parts of the brain?

   cerebrum, cerebellum, brain stem

5. Where in the body is the brain stem?

   in the neck

6. What parts of the body does the brain stem connect to?

   the brain and spinal cord

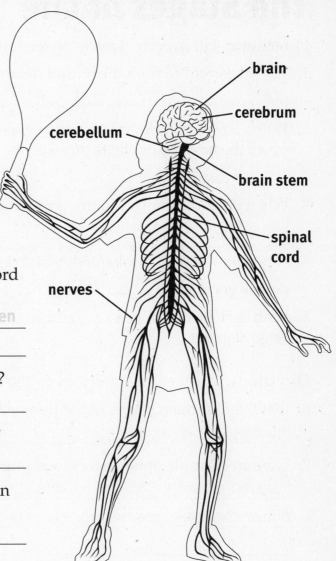

brain

cerebrum

cerebellum

brain stem

spinal cord

nerves

The Stages of Life

Directions: Fill in each blank with the term that matches the description.

1. The stages of life from birth until death make up the _____life cycle_____.

2. When a person feels happy one moment and then upset the next, he or she is probably having a _____mood swing_____.

3. When an adolescent suddenly grows taller, he or she has had a _____growth spurt_____.

4. A person who can think quickly and decide what to do has good _____critical thinking skills_____.

5. With each birthday, you _____age_____, or grow older.

Vocabulary
age
critical thinking skills
growth spurt
life cycle
mood swing

Directions: Answer the questions on the lines provided.

6. List the four main stages in the human life cycle.
   infancy, childhood, adolescence, adulthood

7. Give an example of when a person might use critical thinking skills.
   Possible answers: solving a problem, such as planning a party,
   doing word problems, playing chess, or putting a puzzle together

The Stages of Life

Directions: Complete the lesson outline by filling in the blanks.

Infancy and Childhood

1. The life cycle includes the stages of life between
_____birth_____ and _____death_____.

2. The first stage in the life cycle is _____infancy_____.

3. The three stages of childhood are called _____early_____,
_____middle_____, and _____late_____ childhood.

Adolescence and Adulthood

4. Adolescents go through _____puberty_____, which causes
many changes in all areas of health.

5. The four stages of adulthood are:

   a. _____young adulthood_____, during which many people learn to live
   on their own.

   b. _____first adulthood_____, during which people are often busy
   with jobs and families.

   c. _____second adulthood_____, also called midlife.

   d. _____late adulthood_____, during which many people have retired.

6. The final stage of the life cycle is _____death_____.

7. It is normal to feel _____grief_____ when someone dies.

Healthful Habits for Life

8. The number of years a person can expect to live is his or her
_____life expectancy_____.

9. Six healthful habits that can help you age in a healthful way are:

   a. _____be physically active_____.

   b. _____eat healthful foods_____.

   c. _____get enough rest and sleep_____.

   d. _____keep your body clean_____.

   e. _____protect your skin from the sun_____.

   f. _____avoid tobacco_____.

You Are Unique

Directions: Use the clues to complete the puzzle.

Across

4. A desire to know about or take part in something
5. Something that causes a person to have difficulty learning

Down

1. One of a kind
2. The way a person best gains skills and information
3. Something you have done or seen

Vocabulary
experience
interest
learning disability
learning style
unique

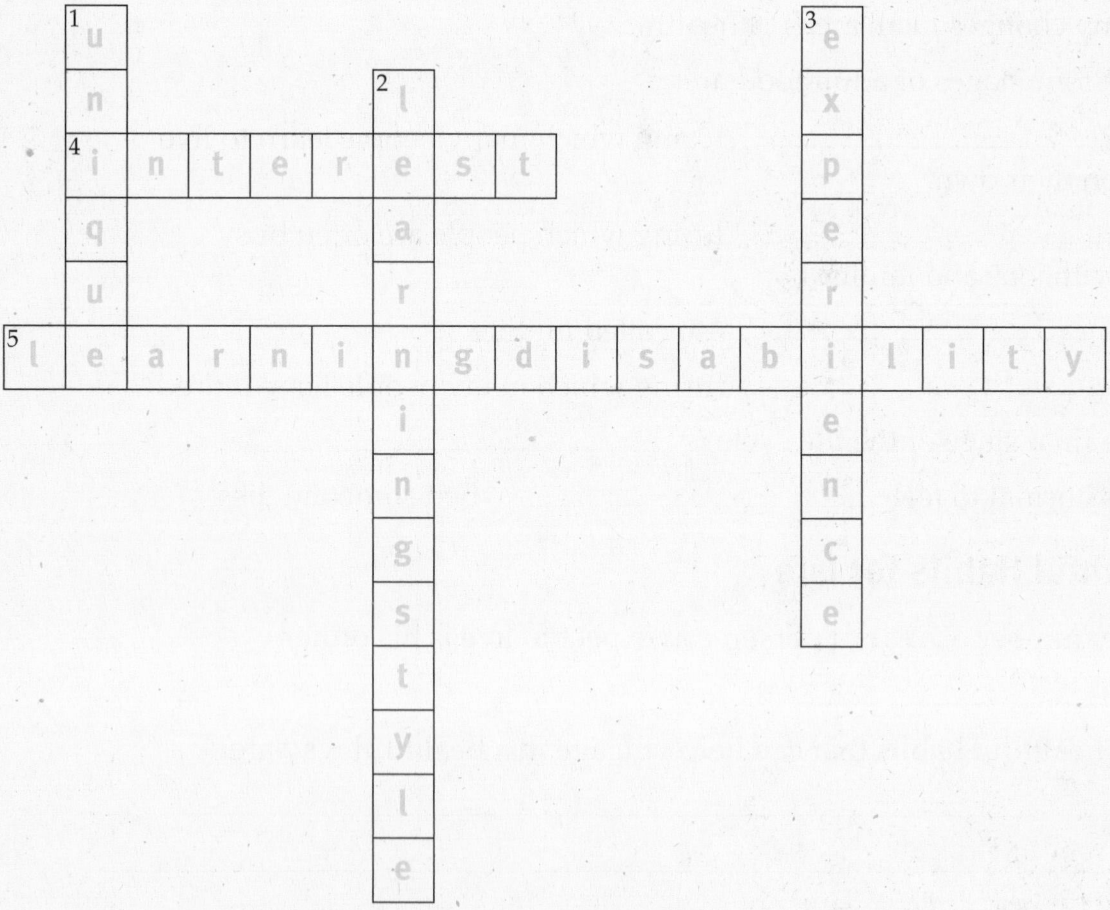

Crossword puzzle:

Down 1: u n i q u e (spelling "unique" with 4 Across crossing)

4 Across: i n t e r e s t

Down 2: l e a r n i n g s t y l e

Down 3: e x p e r i e n c e

5 Across: l e a r n i n g d i s a b i l i t y

You Are Unique

Directions: Complete the lesson outline by filling in the blanks.

Heredity

1. You inherited many traits from your _____birth parents_____.

2. You are _____unique_____ because no one else is exactly like you.

Other Factors

3. Your _____personality_____ is the way you behave and feel.

4. Your experiences are things you have _____seen or done_____.

5. Your _____interests_____ are things you would like to know about or take part in.

6. You keep your _____private thoughts_____ to yourself.

7. The way a person best gain skills and information is his or her _____learning style_____.

8. Some ways to learn are by _____reading_____, _____listening_____, or _____doing_____.

9. Learning and working on projects with other people is called _____cooperative_____ learning.

10. A _____learning disability_____ can cause a person to have difficulty learning.

Practice Healthful Behaviors

Directions: Use these steps to help you outline what you will include in your booklet or brochure. Be sure to give specific tips on how a person can make this behavior a habit. The steps are listed at the right as a reminder.

> 1. Learn about a healthful behavior.
> 2. Practice the behavior.
> 3. Ask for help if you need it.
> 4. Make the behavior a habit.

1. a. What are some healthful behaviors?

Answers will vary.

b. Circle the healthful behavior you want to focus on. What are the health benefits of this behavior? What is important to tell people in your brochure?

Answers will vary.

2. What are some ways that a person can practice this behavior? What tips can you give that will make practicing the behavior easier to remember or do?

Answers will vary.

3. List others who can help a person practice this behavior. Don't forget to suggest asking a parent or guardian for help if needed.

Answers will vary.

4. a. How will a person reading the brochure and putting your tips into action know that he or she has made the behavior a habit? Give some ideas.

Answers will vary.

b. What could the person do if he or she is having trouble forming the habit? Who could he or she go to for help? What else could he or she do?

Answers will vary.

Your Basic Nutritional Needs

Directions: Fill in each blank with the term that matches the description.

1. One medium orange or one slice of bread is an example of a ___serving size___.

2. Hamburgers and eggs are part of the same ___food group___.

3. The ___Dietary Guidelines___ are goals to help you live a healthy life.

4. The smallest slice of ___MyPyramid___ shows that you should eat fats and sweets sparingly.

5. If you eat the recommended amount from each food group, you have a ___balanced diet___.

6. The energy you get from food can be measured in ___calories___.

Vocabulary
balanced diet
calories
Dietary Guidelines
food group
MyPyramid
serving size

Directions: Answer the questions on the lines provided.

7. In what food group would you find tuna fish?
   Meat and Beans Group

8. In what food group would you find oatmeal?
   Grains Group

9. What are the three major parts of the Dietary Guidelines?
   Aim for Fitness, Build a Healthy Base, and Choose Sensibly

10. Explain how MyPyramid can help you plan a balanced diet.
    Possible answer: I can use MyPyramid to find out how much I need from each group to have a balanced diet.

Your Basic Nutritional Needs

Directions: Complete the lesson outline by filling in the blanks.

Six Nutrients You Need

1. The six kinds of nutrients you get from a healthful diet are:
   a. __proteins__ that your body uses to repair cells and to grow.
   b. __carbohydrates__ that are your body's main source of energy.
   c. __fats__ that help store vitamins and supply energy.
   d. __vitamins__ that help fight disease and help body systems work.
   e. __minerals__ that help your body work well and build new cells.
   f. __water__ that your body uses to stay at the right temperature, digest food, and get rid of waste.

MyPyramid

2. A __balanced diet__ includes the correct number of servings from each __food group__.

3. __MyPyramid__ shows how much you need from each food group each day.

4. The five major food groups are the:
   a. __Grains Group__, from which you need 6 oz.
   b. __Vegetable Group__, from which you need 2 1/2 cups
   c. __Fruit Group__, from which you need 1 1/2 cups
   d. __Meat and Beans Group__, from which you need 5 oz.
   e. __Milk Group__, from which you need 3 cups.

5. A balanced diet includes only small amounts of __fats, oils, and sweets__.

continued

continued

The Dietary Guidelines

6. The Dietary Guidelines are suggested _____goals_____ to help you live a long and healthy life.

7. To remember the Dietary Guidelines, you can think of ABC. This stands for:

   a. A ___Aim for Fitness___

   b. B ___Build a Healthy Base___

   c. C ___Choose Sensibly___

8. Two ways to meet the first part of the Dietary Guidelines are:

   a. ___Aim for a healthful weight___.

   b. ___Be physically active each day___.

9. To meet the second part of the Dietary Guidelines, you can:

   a. ___Use MyPyramid to guide your food choices___.

   b. ___Eat a variety of grains daily___.

   c. ___Eat vegetables and fruits daily___.

   d. ___Keep food safe to eat___.

10. To meet the third part of the Dietary Guidelines, limit the ___fat___, ___salt___, and ___sugar___ you eat. Avoid drinking ___alcohol___.

11. Three ways to limit the fat in your diet are:

    a. ___Eat grains, fruits, and vegetables___.

    b. ___Choose fish, poultry, and lean meat___.

    c. ___Avoid fried foods___.

MyPyramid

Directions: MyPyramid shows you how much from each food group you need each day for a balanced diet. Use MyPyramid below to answer the questions.

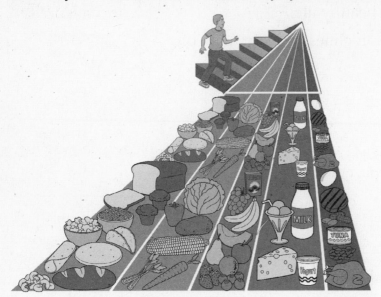

1. What food groups are shown on the diagram?

   Grains Group; Vegetable Group; Fruit Group;

   Meat and Beans Group; Milk Group

2. Which group has the largest slice of the pyramid? What does this mean?

   Grains Group; It means that I should eat the most

   from this group.

3. How much should you eat each day from the Fruit Group?

   $1\frac{1}{2}$ cups

4. Should you eat more from the Vegetable Group or the Meat and Beans Group?

   the Vegetable Group

5. What kinds of foods should you eat only in small amounts?

   Fats, Oils, and Sweets. They have the smallest slice in MyPyramid.

Aim for a Balanced Diet

Directions: Fill in each blank with the term that matches the description.

1. You can find information about the nutrients in a packaged food on the ___Nutrition Facts label___.

2. A(n) ___fast food___ can be cooked quickly and easily and sold to customers.

3. ___MyPyramid___ can help you plan your meals for good nutrition.

4. A food eaten by people from a specific culture is called a(n) ___ethnic food___.

5. When you plan how much food to eat, you should consider the ___portion___.

6. A food made up of foods from more than one food group is a(n) ___combination food___.

Vocabulary
combination food
ethnic food
fast food
MyPyramid
Nutrition Facts label
portion

Directions: Answer the questions on the lines provided.

7. Where on a package of food would you look to find the portion or serving size?

The Nutrition Facts label

8. Suppose you are planning to eat a combination food. What do you need to remember when you plan your meals that day?

To count all the food groups that make up the combination food.

9. How might your family's culture influence your food choices?

Possible answer: There may be an ethnic food we like to eat.

10. How can you use the Nutrition Facts label to help you plan meals?

Possible answer: I can read the label to find out the amount of nutrients in the food, so I can be sure I get enough of the right nutrients.

Aim for a Balanced Diet

Directions: Complete the lesson outline by filling in the blanks.

Influences on Food Choices

1. Six things that can influence your food choices are:

   a. personal preferences .   d. advertising .

   b. family and peers .   e. cost and availability .

   c. emotions .   f. health benefits .

Meals and Snacks

2. Two tools you can use to help plan what you will eat are MyPyramid and the Dietary Guidelines .

3.

Food	Serving Size
a. Cooked cereal, rice, or pasta	$\frac{1}{2}$ cup, or about the size of an ice cream scoop
Cheese	b. 2 ounces, or about the size of 2 dominoes
Vegetables	c. 1 cup, or about the size of an adult's fist

4. A combination food has servings from more than one food group.

5. A fast food can be cooked and served quickly.

Food Labels

6. The Nutrition Facts label can give you information about the nutrients in a food. It also tells you about nutrients you should limit, such as fat and sodium .

Serving Sizes

Directions: When you plan your meals, it's important to know how much of a food you should eat. Use the chart to answer the questions.

1. What does this chart show?

The names of foods and information about amounts for the foods

2. What is one serving of dry cereal? What does this amount look like?

One cup; it is about the amount that can be held in a hand.

3. For which food is 2 ounces a serving size? What does this amount look like?

Cheese; it looks like two dominoes.

4. Is a serving of peanut butter larger or smaller than a serving of meat?

smaller

5. Which is the smallest serving size? Why do you think that is?

Butter; fats should be used only in small amounts because they are

high in calories.

Amounts for Different Foods				
Food	**Amount**	**Food**	**Amount**
$\frac{1}{2}$ cup cooked cereal, rice, or pasta 1 cup dry cereal	ice cream scoop palm of hand	2 ounces cheese	2 dominos
1 cup cut vegetables	fist	2 tablespoons peanut butter	ping pong ball
1 medium-sized piece of fruit	baseball	2–3 ounces meat	palm of adult hand
		1 teaspoon butter	adult thumb

Name   Date

Food Labels

Directions: Knowing how to read food labels can help you plan healthful meals. Use this label to answer the questions.

1. Where would you find this label?

   on a food package

2. What information would you find in section A?

   the serving size or amount

   and number of servings

3. Where would you look to find the amount of protein in

   the food? _____section E_____

4. Which section shows information about nutrients you should limit? Which nutrients are these?

   section D; saturated fats, cholesterol,

   trans fats, cholesterol, and sodium

5. What information is not shown on this label that you might want to look at when you choose a food?

   Possible information: the list

   of ingredients

Nutrition Facts

Serving Size 1 cup (228g) **A**
Serving Per Container 2

Amount Per Serving

Calories 80 **B**   Calories from Fat 20

	% Daily Value*
Total Fat 4g **D**	**6%**
Saturated Fat 3g	**15%**
Trans Fat 1g	
Cholesterol 10mg	**3%**
Sodium 390mg **D**	**16%**
Total Carbohydrate 17g **E**	**6%**
Dietary Fiber 4g	**16%**
Sugars 8g	
Protein 6g **E**	

Vitamin A	140%
Vitamin C	25%
Calcium	4%
Iron	10%

*Percent Daily Values are based on a 2,000 calorie diet. Your Daily Values may be higher or lower depending on your calorie needs. **C**

	Calories:	2,000	2,500
Total Fat	Less than	65g	80g
Sat Fat	Less than	20g	25g
Cholesterol	Less than	300mg	300mg
Sodium	Less than	2,400mg	2,400mg
Total Carbohydrate	**F**	300g	375g
Dietary Fiber		25g	30g

Analyze What Influences Your Health

Directions: In a grocery store, choose a food that comes in a package that you think is attractive. Analyze why it appeals to you and how it might influence your health.

1. Why does the package appeal to me?

   Possible answers: It uses bright colors,

   it has a picture of a sports star I like on it, it

   offers a free toy if I buy it

2. If I bought this product, how could it affect my health?

   Students' answers should reflect an

   understanding of whether the product

   is a healthful food or not and how eating

   it could affect their health.

3. How could the packaging influence me to make a healthful choice?

   Students should discuss analyzing the Nutrition Facts panel,

   ingredients list, or other statements that provide information on the

   healthfulness of the food.

4. How could the packaging influence me to make a harmful choice?

   Students' answers should show understanding

   that the use of flashy packaging, celebrity endorsements,

   and so on could lead them to ignore health information.

> **Analyze What Influences Your Health**
>
> 1. Identify people and things that can influence your health.
> 2. Evaluate how these people and things can affect your health.
> 3. Choose healthful influences.
> 4. Protect yourself against harmful influences.

Food That's Safe to Eat

Directions: Write the letter of the correct answer on the line.

___D___ 1. Safe and polite ways to eat

___A___ 2. A way to help someone who is choking

___B___ 3. Caused by eating food or drinking a beverage that is contaminated

___C___ 4. A germ that causes disease

Vocabulary
A abdominal thrust
B foodborne illness
C pathogen
D table manners

Directions: Explain how table manners can help with food safety and make meals more pleasant.

5. Possible answer: Washing my hands before I eat lowers the risk of some illnesses. Using a napkin protects me from spills. Taking small bites and eating slowly helps keep me from choking. These all help with food safety. Waiting my turn, sharing food, and eating in pleasant ways can make the meal more pleasant because these behaviors show respect for myself and others.

Food That's Safe to Eat

Directions: Complete the lesson outline by filling in the blanks.

How Pathogens Enter Food

1. A _____pathogen_____ is a germ that causes disease.

2. Three ways that pathogens can enter food while it is grown and processed are:

   a. _Water can spread pathogens to plants or animals_.

   b. _Workers who do not wash their hands can spread pathogens to food_.

   c. _Food may contact pathogens on surfaces_.

Safety Guidelines for Food

3. Four major ways to keep food safe are:

   a. _wash hands, foods, and utensils_.

   b. _store and prepare foods separately_.

   c. _cook raw food properly_.

   d. _keep some foods cold_.

Table Manners

4. Three table manners that can help keep you safe are:

   a. _washing your hands before you eat_.

   b. _putting a napkin in your lap to protect from spills_.

   c. _eating slowly and taking small bites to avoid choking_.

5. A(n) _____abdominal thrust_____ is a way to help a person who is choking.

Your Weight Manager

Directions: Fill in each blank with the term that matches the description.

1. A person who weighs less than his or her healthful weight is __underweight__.

2. A(n) __eating disorder__ is a harmful way of eating because a person cannot cope with a situation.

3. Your __body image__ is how you feel about the way you look.

4. A(n) __weight management__ plan helps you have a healthful weight.

5. A person who weighs more than his or her healthful weight is __overweight__.

6. The best weight for your body is a(n) __healthful weight__.

Vocabulary
body image
eating disorder
healthful weight
overweight
underweight
weight management

Directions: Answer the questions on the lines provided.

7. If you take in about as many calories as you use, what will happen to your weight?
   It will remain about the same.

8. If a person is overweight, what might he or she do to reach a desirable weight?
   Use more calories than he or she takes in.

9. Give three examples of eating disorders.
   binge eating disorder, bulimia nervosa, anorexia nervosa

10. How do you feel when you have a positive body image?
    Possible answer: You like and accept how your body looks.

Your Weight Manager

Directions: Complete the lesson outline by filling in the blanks.

A Healthful Weight

1. You can use ___weight management___ to have a
    healthful weight.

2. If you use the same number of calories as you eat, your
    weight will ___stay about the same___.

Weighing In

3. Eating more calories than you use leads to being
    ___overweight___. Eating fewer calories than you
    use leads to being ___underweight___.

4. Being overweight increases the risk of:

    a. ___heart disease___.

    b. ___diabetes___.

    c. ___some kinds of cancer___.

Body Image

5. Your body image is the feeling you have about
    ___the way your body looks___.

6. Some people develop ___eating disorders___ because
    they cannot cope with a situation.

    Three examples of these are:

    a. ___binge eating disorder___, in which a person eats too
        much all at once.

    b. ___bulimia nervosa___, in which a person eats a lot of
        food and then tries to get rid of it.

    c. ___anorexia nervosa___, in which a person eats very little or
        nothing at all.

Calorie Chart

Directions: The chart lists the calories in some foods. It also lists the calories burned by several kinds of physical activity. Use the chart to answer the questions.

Calories in Food			Calories Used by a 100-Pound Person	
Food	**Portion**	**Number of Calories**	**Activity**	**Calories Used per hour**
Broccoli (cooked)	1 cup	44	Swimming slowly	about 195
Bread (wheat)	1 slice	65	Bicycling (12 miles per hour)	about 290
Egg	1 large	75	Walking (3 miles per hour)	about 225
Blueberries	1 cup	81	Swimming fast	about 350
Low-fat milk	1 cup	102	Jumping rope	about 525
Skinless chicken breast (roasted)	3 oz.	142	Running (10 miles per hour)	about 900

1. How many calories are in one cup of cooked broccoli?

   44

2. Where would you look to find out how many calories are burned by jumping rope? the last column of the fifth row

3. Juanita weighs about 100 pounds. For dinner, she ate three ounces of skinless chicken breast, a slice of bread, one cup of broccoli, and one cup of low-fat milk. What activity could she do to use the calories she ate? How long would she need to do the activity?

   Possible answer: Swimming fast for about one hour

Caring for Your Body

Directions: Use the clues to complete the puzzle.

Across

5. Taking care of your body and appearance
7. A series of tests that measure your health status

Down

1. A lotion or cream that blocks the sun's harmful rays
2. The steps your body goes through during sleep
3. A curving of the spine to one side of the body
4. The way you hold your body as you sit, stand, and move
6. The stage of sleep when you dream
8. A skin disorder in which clogged pores become inflamed, or swollen

Vocabulary

acne

grooming

medical checkup

posture

REM

scoliosis

sleep cycle

sunscreen

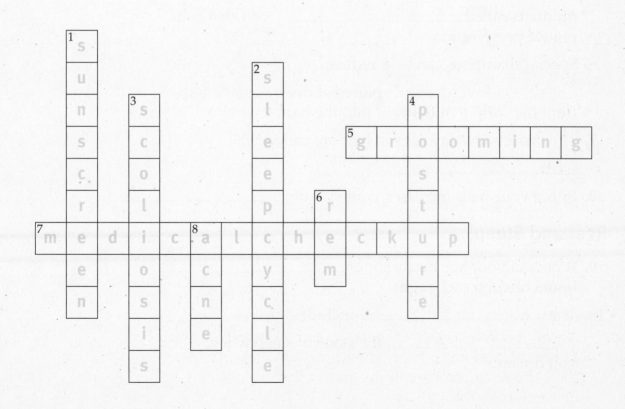

Caring for Your Body

Directions: Complete the lesson outline by filling in the blanks.

Medical Checkups

1. Getting a _____medical checkup_____ at least once a year is important to make sure your body is working well.

2. Having good _____posture_____ helps your skeletal and muscular systems.

Good Grooming

3. You can help protect your skin from the sun by wearing _____sunscreen_____.

4. Washing your face every day can help reduce the skin disorder _____acne_____.

5. Grooming products called _____deodorants_____ help control odor under your arms. Other grooming products called _____antiperspirants_____ can also help reduce perspiration.

6. Special shampoos can help reduce _____dandruff_____, pieces of dry or greasy skin from the scalp that flake off into the hair.

7. Tiny insects that lay eggs in hair are called _____head lice_____.

8. Biting your nails increases your risk of _____illness_____.

Rest and Sleep

9. A person your age needs about _____ten_____ hours of sleep each night.

10. The _____sleep cycle_____ includes _____REM_____, the stage of sleep when you dream.

Your Skin

Directions: Your skin is the largest organ of your body. Washing your skin every day is an important part of good grooming and helps to keep your skin healthy. Use the diagram to answer the questions on the lines provided. Use complete sentences.

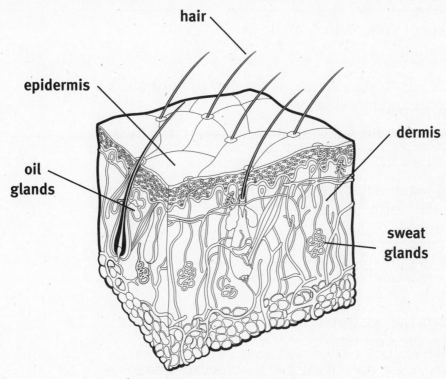

1. Compare and contrast the epidermis and the dermis.

   The epidermis is thinner and is the outer layer of skin. The dermis is
   thicker and is the inner layer of skin. The dermis contains the structures
   of the skin.

2. Which structures are located in the dermis?

   The skin structures located in the dermis are the oil glands and the
   sweat glands.

3. How do sweat and oil reach the skin's surface?

   Sweat and oil reach the skin's surface through pores.

4. When you wash your face, which layer of the skin are you washing?

   You wash the epidermis when you wash your face.

Your Teeth, Eyes, and Ears

Directions: Use the words below to fill in the blanks.

cavities	dental plaque	enamel	lens
periodontal disease	pulp	pupil	retina

1. The surface of your teeth is made of
   _____enamel_____.

2. The _____pulp_____ is the part of your tooth that holds nerves and blood vessels.

3. The sticky substance on teeth that contains bacteria is called _____dental plaque_____.

4. If dental plaque is not removed from teeth, it combines with sugar to form an acid that can cause _____cavities_____.

5. A disease of the gums and bone that support the teeth is called _____periodontal disease_____.

6. Light enters the eye through the_____pupil_____, a hole in the eye's center.

7. The curved, clear part of the eye that focuses images is called the _____lens_____.

8. The _____retina_____ sends messages from the eye to the brain.

Directions: Write the letter of the correct answer on the line.

Vocabulary	
A	audiologist
B	cochlea
C	decibel
D	ear canal
E	eardrum
F	hearing loss

____B____ 9. The shell-shaped part of the ear that is filled with fluid

____F____ 10. The inability to hear or interpret certain sounds

____D____ 11. The part of the ear that carries sound to your eardrum

____C____ 12. A unit used to measure the loudness of sound

____E____ 13. The thin membrane that vibrates when hit by sound

____A____ 14. A hearing specialist

Your Teeth, Eyes, and Ears

Directions: Complete the lesson outline by filling in the blanks.

Your Teeth

1. The surface of teeth is made of _____ enamel _____.

2. Dental plaque contains _____ bacteria _____.

3. Cavities can form if dental plaque combines with _____ sugar _____.

4. Brushing and flossing your teeth every day removes _____ dental plaque _____ and helps prevent _____ periodontal disease _____.

Your Eyes

5. Habits you can use to keep your eyes healthy are:
   a. Get a yearly vision check.
   b. Read or watch television in well-lit areas.
   c. Rest the eyes every few minutes when using a computer.
   d. Do not rub eyes if they itch or burn. Tell a parent or guardian.
   e. Wear sunglasses.
   f. Wear safety glasses when you play sports that require them.
   g. Never run with or throw anything sharp or pointed.

Your Ears

6. A hearing specialist called an _____ audiologist _____ may test a person's ears for _____ hearing loss _____.

7. To protect your ears and hearing:
   a. Never put anything in your ears.
   b. Tell a parent or guardian if your ear aches.
   c. Avoid loud sounds.

Vision Problems

Directions: Some people have trouble seeing things close up or far away. This happens because their eyes are an irregular shape. Use the drawings to answer the questions on the lines provided.

Normal Eye   **Nearsighted Eye**   **Farsighted Eye**

lens   lens   lens

pupil   pupil   pupil

retina   retina   retina

1. On which part of the eye should an image be focused in order for a person to see normally?

   The image should be focused on the retina.

2. Where is the image focused in a person who is nearsighted?

   In a person who is nearsighted, the image is focused in front of the retina.

3. Where is the image focused in a person who is farsighted?

   In a person who is farsighted, the image is focused behind the retina.

4. What problems might a person who is farsighted experience trying to read a book?

   The words would likely be blurry.

5. Describe the shape of the eye in a person who is nearsighted. How might this shape be different from the shape of the eye in a person with normal vision?

   A nearsighted person's eyeball is elongated compared to a normal person's eyeball. The lens in a nearsighted person's eyeball may be thicker.

The Benefits of Physical Activity

Directions: Write the letter of the correct answer on the line.

		Vocabulary

_C_ 1. Skills that can be used during physical activities

_D_ 2. Having your heart, lungs, muscles, and joints in top condition

_B_ 3. The amount of blood pumped by your heart each minute

_A_ 4. The force of blood against artery walls

Vocabulary

A blood pressure

B cardiac output

C fitness skills

D health fitness

Directions: Use the words below to fill in the blanks.

heart rate	fitness skills	blood pressure
President's Challenge	health fitness	flexibility

5. A test sponsored by the government that measures your level of physical fitness is the ___President's Challenge___.

6. The number of times your heart beats each minute is your ___heart rate___.

7. Agility, coordination, and power are all examples of ___fitness skills___.

8. High ___blood pressure___ harms the arteries.

9. Muscular endurance, flexibility, and body composition are all examples of ___health fitness___.

10. The ability to bend and move your body easily is ___flexibility___.

The Benefits of Physical Activity

Directions: Complete the lesson outline by filling in the blanks.

Physical Fitness

1. Having your body in top condition is
   <u>physical fitness</u>.

Health Fitness

2. The five kinds of health fitness are:

   a. <u>cardiorespiratory endurance</u>

   b. <u>muscular endurance</u>

   c. <u>flexibility</u>

   d. <u>body composition</u>

   e. <u>muscular strength</u>

Test Your Skills

3. The six major fitness skills are:

   a. <u>agility</u>

   b. <u>balance</u>

   c. <u>coordination</u>

   d. <u>reaction time</u>

   e. <u>speed</u>

   f. <u>power</u>

4. An example of a test that measures your physical fitness
   and fitness skills is the <u>President's Challenge</u>.

Name　　　　　　　　　　**Date**

A Balanced Workout

Directions: Write the letter of the correct answer on the line.

_C_　**1.** The gradual increase in overload necessary to achieve higher levels of fitness

_B_　**2.** Working your body harder than normal to improve your health fitness

_E_　**3.** A fast and safe heart rate for workouts

_A_　**4.** How often something happens

_D_　**5.** Doing specific exercises and activities to improve particular areas of fitness

_F_　**6.** Doing specific exercises to improve a particular fitness skill or type of health fitness

Vocabulary
A frequency
B overload
C progression
D specificity
E target heart rate
F training

Directions: Answer the questions on the lines provided.

7. You want to improve the muscle strength in your arms, so you do push-ups and pull-ups as part of your workout.

This is an example of _____specificity_____.

8. Give an example of how to use progression to achieve a higher level of fitness. __Increase the frequency, intensity, or amount of time spent doing an activity.__

9. How could increasing the frequency of your workouts affect your strength and endurance?
__It would improve them.__

10. By exercising at a level that maintains your target heart rate, you can build your ____cardiorespiratory endurance____.

A Balanced Workout

Directions: Complete the lesson outline by filling in the blanks.

Benefits of Physical Activity

1. To plan specific physical activities to reach a physical
   fitness goal is to _____ exercise _____.

2. How hard you work during exercise is described as
   _____ intensity _____.

3. There are three levels of intensity:

   a. _____ low _____

   b. _____ moderate _____

   c. _____ vigorous _____

4. To be physically fit, get _____ 60 _____ minutes
   of _____ moderate _____-intensity physical activity each
   day. Get _____ 30 _____ minutes of
   _____ vigorous _____-intensity physical activity 3–4
   times a week.

Getting Started

5. Before you begin to exercise, check with your
   _____ parent or guardian _____ and get a _____ medical checkup _____.

6. During _____ aerobic _____ exercise you use large
   amounts of oxygen over a long time. _____ Walking, jogging,
   bicycling, swimming and in-line skating _____
   are examples of this type of exercise.

7. Exercises that use short periods of hard work
   followed by periods of rest are _____ anaerobic _____
   exercises. These exercises improve your muscle
   _____ strength and endurance _____.

continued

continued

8. Choose a _____variety_____ of physical
   activities to improve your _____health fitness_____
   and _____fitness skills_____.

Work Out

9. Each exercise session should consist of three parts:
   a. ____warm-up____
   b. ____workout____
   c. ____cool-down____

10. Before exercising, _____warming up_____ helps prevent injuries.

11. A fast, safe heart rate for workouts is your _____target heart rate_____.

12. Specificity, training, overload, frequency, and _____progression_____ are all part of exercising to improve your health fitness or fitness skills.

13. The acronym FITT stands for:
    a. F ____frequency____
    b. I ____intensity____
    c. T ____time____
    d. T ____type____

14. Five to ten minutes of easy physical activity done after a workout is called a _____cool-down_____.

Setting Health Goals for Fitness

15. Your age, _____heredity_____, and level of fitness affect your fitness needs.

16. In order to work out every day, you need to make _____time_____ in your schedule.

Name   Date

Play It Safe

Directions: Write the letter of the correct answer on the line.

_D_ **1.** An injury to the tissue that connects bones to a joint

_C_ **2.** Treatment used for sprains and other injuries to muscles and bones

_B_ **3.** Rules that say what equipment must be made of and how it must work

_A_ **4.** An overstretch of a muscle

Vocabulary
A muscle strain
B safety equipment standards
C PRICE
D sprain

Directions: Fill in each numbered blank in the table with the correct term or phrase.

P	Protect	5. Use an elastic bandage, splint, or sling to protect the injured area.
R	6. Rest	Stop using the injured arm or leg right away.
I	Ice	7. Put ice on the area.
C	Compression	8. Wrap the injured area in a soft bandage.
E	9. Elevation	Raise the injured area to a level above the heart.

Play It Safe

Directions: Complete the lesson outline by filling in the blanks.

Safety in Sports and Games

1. Safety equipment can help reduce your risk of ___injury___.

2. Safety equipment should meet ___safety equipment standards___.

A Safe Workout

3. Before physical activity:
   a. ___Choose proper clothing and safety equipment.___
   b. ___Make sure equipment is in order.___
   c. ___Warm up.___
   d. ___Drink water.___

4. During physical activity:
   a. ___Drink more water.___
   b. ___Keep track of your heart rate.___
   c. ___Rest or stop if you think you have an injury.___

5. After physical activity:
   a. ___Cool down.___
   b. ___Check your heart rate.___
   c. ___Continue to drink water.___

6. Two common injuries are muscle ___strains___ and ___sprains___.

Be a Good Sport

7. A ___good sport___ plays fair, ___respects___ others, and follows ___rules___.

8. If you lose a competition, keep a ___positive attitude___.

Access Health Products

Directions: Decide what safety equipment you need to play a sport of your choice. To help you make your decision, answer the questions on the lines provided using complete sentences. The steps for accessing health products are listed to the right to help you as you work.

<table>
<tr><td colspan="2">Access Health Products</td></tr>
<tr><td>1.</td><td>Identify when you might need health products.</td></tr>
<tr><td>2.</td><td>Identify where you might find health products.</td></tr>
<tr><td>3.</td><td>Find the health products you need.</td></tr>
<tr><td>4.</td><td>Evaluate the health products.</td></tr>
</table>

1. What sport do you want to investigate? What equipment does this sport require?

   Students' sport choices will vary.

   _____

2. Where can you purchase the equipment you need? Where can you find information about safety standards for the equipment?

   Safety equipment can be purchased at specialty sports equipment

   stores, from the sports section of a department store, from a catalog,

   or on the Internet. Information on safety standards for the equipment

   should be available on equipment labels, in a catalog or the library,

   or on the Internet.

3. With your parents or guardian, go to a store or look at a catalog. Write down the information you learn.

   Students should decide which product(s) they may be interested in

   buying based on safety, durability, fit, quality, and cost.

4. Based on the information you have found, which product would you buy? Why?

   Information they found about safety, durability, fit, quality, and cost should

   help them make a decision about which product to purchase.

Name   **Date**

Keep Safe Indoors

Directions: Match the correct letter with the description.

_____E____ **1.** A device that sounds an alarm when smoke
is present

_____B____ **2.** Something that can cause harm or injury

_____D____ **3.** Guidelines to help prevent injury

_____A____ **4.** A device containing water or chemicals to spray
on a fire

_____C____ **5.** Harm done to a person

Vocabulary
A fire extinguisher
B hazard
C injury
D safety rules
E smoke detector

Directions: Answer the questions on the lines provided.

6. List three examples of common hazards at home
that can cause harm.

Possible answers: toys on stairs, wet floor, an old furnace leaking

carbon monoxide

7. Why is a smoke detector helpful?

It sounds an alarm when smoke is present.

8. Name three types of injury that can be avoided at home
and an example of how to avoid each of them.

Possible answers: accidental poisoning: keep cleaners and medicines

in separate cabinets; burns: turn pan handles toward the center of the

stove; falls: keep floors clear

9. Name four hazards that you should watch out for in
school and at playgrounds.

Possible answers: School—water on floors, debris in halls or aisles;

Playgrounds—broken equipment, hard surfaces beneath equipment

10. How can you avoid the danger of inhaling smoke during
a fire?

Crawl on your hands and knees to stay beneath the smoke.

Keep Safe Indoors

Directions: Complete the lesson outline by filling in the blanks.

Safety at Home

1. Accidents at home can cause _____injury_____, or harm, to a person.

2. A scraped knee is a minor injury. However if a person gets a _____serious_____ injury, he or she may need to get extra care.

3. Three ways you can reduce hazards in your home are

   a. keep floors _____clear_____ so that people don't trip and fall.

   b. keep _____cleaners and medicines_____ in separate cabinets where _____small children_____ can't reach them.

   c. don't use electrical items when you are _____wet_____.

4. You can reduce the risk of injury by following _____safety_____ rules.

Fire Safety

5. Fire _____extinguishers_____ and _____smoke detectors_____ can help to protect your home if there is a fire.

6. With your family, you can _____plan_____ how to get out if there is a fire.

7. You can help prevent fires by using the following safety rules.

   a. Turn pan handles toward the _____center_____ of the stove.

   b. Use _____potholders_____ when you move a hot pan.

   c. Never play with _____matches_____; you could accidentally start a fire.

   d. Make sure that electrical cords don't run under _____rugs_____.

   e. Don't plug too many appliances into one _____outlet_____.

   f. Don't leave _____appliances_____ running with no one nearby.

continued

continued

8. You and your family can practice what to do in case of fire by having _____fire drills_____.

9. You should know _____two_____ ways to get out of a room in case _____one way is blocked_____ in a fire.

10. In the case of fire, _____yell loudly_____ to alert others.

11. In a fire, if a door feels hot, _____don't open it_____.

12. If there is smoke, _____crawl on your hands and knees_____ to stay below the level of _____smoke_____ so that you don't _____breathe_____ it.

13. After you get out, _____meet your family_____ outside.

Safety at School

14. Four ways you can stay safe at school are

   a. keep the hallways and _____aisles_____ in your school clear.

   b. don't _____run_____ in hallways.

   c. don't _____push_____ anyone else, especially someone drinking from a _____water fountain_____.

   d. if you see a wet floor, tell a _____teacher_____.

15. On a playground, only use equipment that is safe and not _____broken_____.

16. Make sure that the ground under playground equipment has a thick layer of _____soft_____ material, such as sand.

17. Always play with a _____friend_____ when playing outside.

18. Always tell a _____parent or guardian_____ where you will be playing

Smoke Detectors

Directions: Use the diagram to answer the questions on the lines provided.

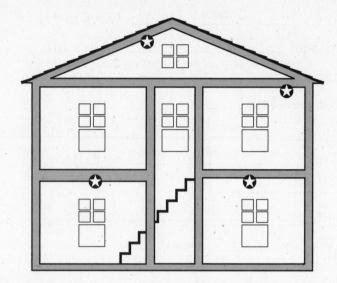

Put smoke detectors on every level of your home. One should be placed near every bedroom. Test the batteries regularly. Change dead batteries right away.

1. What does the diagram show?

   It shows where to install smoke detectors in a house.

2. What are two important rules to remember when deciding where to put smoke detectors in your home?

   Put smoke detectors on every level.

   Put one detector near every bedroom.

3. What part of a smoke detector should you test and change regularly?

   the battery

4. How do you think smoke detectors help people in a home?

   They alert people to the presence of smoke in the air.

5. In addition to smoke detectors, what other type of detector can prevent injury from a faulty furnace?

   carbon monoxide detector

Keep Safe Outdoors

Directions: Match the correct letter with the description.

_D_ **1.** The lap belt and shoulder belt worn in a car that keep you from being thrown from the car in the case of an accident

_B_ **2.** Harm to the body due to being exposed to high temperatures

_C_ **3.** A person who walks on the sidewalk or in the street

_A_ **4.** An injury caused by exposure to extreme cold

Vocabulary
A frostbite
B heatstroke
C pedestrian
D seat belt

Directions: Fill in the blanks in the chart below.

What to Do for Heatstroke and Frostbite		
Name of Injury	**What to Look For**	**What to Do**
Heatstroke	**5.** • A very <u>high temperature</u>. • Skin that is hot and dry.	**6.** • Get the person in the shade right away. • Use <u>water</u> to cool the body.
Frostbite	**7.** • Skin that is numb. • Skin that is <u>white, gray, or yellow</u>.	**8.** • Get the person into a <u>warm room</u>. • Get medical help right away.

9. List two safety rules for pedestrians.

Possible answers: use sidewalks and crosswalks, obey traffic signals, walk facing traffic if there are no sidewalks, wear light-colored clothes if you are out in the dark, walk with a friend, don't hitchhike.

10. What should you do if an adult you do not know asks you for directions or to help find a lost pet?

Possible answers: Say "No!" in a loud, firm voice, run in the opposite direction from the person or his or her car, and tell a parent or other responsible adult what happened.

Keep Safe Outdoors

Directions: Complete the lesson outline by filling in the blanks.

Walk Safely

1. A person who walks on the sidewalk or in the street is called a ___pedestrian___.

2. Follow these five safety rules when you walk outdoors.

   a. Use ___crosswalks___ and ___sidewalks___. Don't enter the street between ___parked cars___

   b. Obey ___traffic signals___. Wait for the ___"Walk"___ sign.

   c. When walking on a street with no sidewalks, walk ___facing___ the traffic.

   d. Wear ___light___-colored or ___reflective___ clothes if you are outside at dusk or at night.

   e. Walk with a ___friend___ or a responsible adult.

3. When ___crossing___ a street, look left, and right, then ___left___ again before you start to cross.

Safe on the Road

4. In a car, people aged 12 or younger should ride in the ___back___ seat to avoid being injured by air bags.

5. When you get off a school bus and need to cross the street, cross ___in front of___ the bus.

6. Whenever you ride in a school bus, ___sit still___ and don't ___yell___ or ___fight___.

7. Wear a ___helmet___ when riding a ___bicycle___, scooter, skates, or skateboards.

8. Wear ___elbow___ and ___knee___ pads and ___wrist___ guards along with a ___helmet___ when you skate or ride a skateboard.

9. When you ride a bicycle, use ___hand___ signals before you ___turn___ or ___stop___.

continued

continued

Weather and Water

10. Very _____hot_____ and very _____cold_____
    weather can cause injuries. Many people are also injured
    when _____swimming_____ and boating.

11. In cold weather, wear several layers of _____clothes_____.

12. If you see a person with signs of frostbite, get the person
    into a _____warm room_____. Get _____medical_____ help
    right away.

13. Follow these suggestions to protect yourself in hot weather.

    a. Drink extra _____water_____.

    b. Wear _____sunscreen_____, a _____hat_____, and
    _____sunglasses_____ to protect yourself from the sun.

    c. If you get sunburned, run _____cool water_____ over the burn.

14. Harm to the body due to being exposed to high
    temperatures is _____heatstroke_____.

15. Symptoms of heatstroke include _____hot, dry skin_____ and a
    very _____high temperature_____.

16. If you see a person with symptoms of heatstroke, get him
    or her into the _____shade_____ right away.

17. If you feel you may have heatstroke, use _____water_____
    to cool your body.

18. Learn how to _____swim_____ to feel more comfortable
    in the water.

19. Never swim _____alone_____. Make sure that _____an adult_____
    is nearby.

20. When you are near water, don't _____run_____ or _____push_____
    other people. You could _____knock someone into the water_____.

21. Never _____dive_____ into any lake or river. The water
    may be _____shallow_____ or have hidden _____rocks_____.

Rules for Walking

Directions: Answer the questions on the lines provided.

1. What does the picture show?

   The picture shows two pedestrians
   walking down a sidewalk at dusk wearing
   light-colored clothes.

2. Why should someone wear light-colored clothing when walking at dusk or after dark?

   Wearing light-colored clothing makes it
   easier for drivers to see a person walking
   at dusk or after dark.

3. Why is crossing a street at a crosswalk safer than crossing between parked cars?

   Crossing at a crosswalk is safer because
   drivers expect to see pedestrians at crosswalks.
   Drivers are less prepared to stop if a pedestrian suddenly
   steps into the street from between parked cars.

4. Why should you never hitchhike?

   You should never hitchhike because getting into a stranger's car
   can be very dangerous.

5. Why is walking with a friend or adult a good idea?

   Doing so will discourage strangers from approaching you.

How to Handle Emergencies

Directions: Match the correct letter with the description.

____F____ 1. An electrical storm than can bring heavy rain, thunder, and lightning

____C____ 2. Sudden flow of water often caused by heavy rains

____G____ 3. Fast-moving, funnel-shaped cloud of wind

____B____ 4. A situation in which help is needed quickly

____E____ 5. A tropical storm with heavy rain and wind

____A____ 6. A shaking or trembling of the ground

____D____ 7. The overflow of water onto normally dry land

Vocabulary
A earthquake
B emergency
C flash flood
D flood
E hurricane
F thunderstorm
G tornado

Directions: Fill in the blanks in the chart below.

Keep Safe in a Natural Disaster		
Natural Disaster	**What It Is**	**How to Keep Safe**
8. Earthquake	A shaking or trembling of the ground	• Drop to the floor. • Get under a sturdy table. • Move away from buildings and electrical wires if outdoors.
9. Flood	The overflow of water onto normally dry land	• Never swim or ride in a car through flood waters. • If you are outside, climb to higher ground.
10. Hurricane	A tropical storm with heavy rain and wind	• Stay indoors. • Stay away from windows.

How to Handle Emergencies

Directions: Complete the lesson outline by filling in the blanks.

What Is an Emergency?

1. If a person gets a deep cut and the cut won't stop
   bleeding, this is an _____emergency_____ and the
   person needs medical help.

2. Decide if each situation is an emergency or not.
   Write *yes* or *no* in the blanks.

   a. a person is having a heart attack ____yes____

   b. someone gets a small cut ____no____

   c. a person has stopped breathing ____yes____

3. A _____terrorist_____ is a person who uses violence
   to try to make another person do what he or she wants.

4. If you think someone has been poisoned, you should call
   _____poison control_____ and say ____where you are____ and
   _____what happened_____.

5. In the case of a serious injury, you should call
   _____9-1-1 or your local emergency number_____.

Planning Ahead

6. You can prepare for an emergency by working with your
   family to make a _____plan of what you will do_____.

7. Four things your family plan should include are

   a. a _____disaster kit_____

   b. a list of _____phone numbers_____

   c. a plan to _____find each other_____ after the emergency is over.

   d. an _____escape_____ plan to get out of the house.

8. In some emergencies, such as storms, there may be a loss of
   _____electricity_____.

continued

continued

9. List five items you might put in a disaster kit.

    a. A _____first aid kit_____ to help treat injuries.

    b. A _____flashlight_____ to help you see if there is no electricity.

    c. A battery-operated _____radio_____ to hear emergency information.

    d. Some _____extra blankets and sheets or clothing_____ to stay warm and comfortable.

    e. Some _____matches in a waterproof container_____ to be able to start a fire for warmth or cooking.

Natural Disasters

10. Storms, floods, and earthquakes are all examples of _____natural disasters_____.

11. Follow these guidelines during a thunderstorm.

    a. Stay away from _____doors and windows_____.

    b. Don't _____take a bath_____ or shower.

    c. Don't talk _____on the phone_____.

    d. Don't use _____electrical appliances_____.

12. Protect yourself from a hurricane by:

    a. boarding up _____windows and doors_____ with wood.

    b. staying _____indoors_____ and away from _____windows_____.

    c. _____evacuating_____ if officials tell you to do so.

13. If you are outdoors during a tornado and can't find shelter, _____lie flat_____ in a ditch or low-lying area.

14. In a flood, never _____swim_____ or _____ride in a car_____ through floodwaters.

15. If you are inside during an earthquake, you should _____drop_____ to the floor and get under a _____sturdy table or desk_____.

16. If you are outdoors during an earthquake, try to move away from _____buildings_____ and _____electrical wires_____.

How to Handle Emergencies

How to Report an Emergency		
Type of Emergency	**Who to Call**	**What to Say**
Fire	9-1-1 or your local emergency number for fire	Say where the fire is and whether anyone is trapped inside.
Serious injury or medical problem	9-1-1 or your local emergency number for medical emergencies	Say where you are. Describe as much about the problem as you can.
Criminal acts or violence	Police or 9-1-1 if the crime is taking place now	Say where you are and what is happening.
Poisoning	Poison Control	Say where you are and what happened. If you have the poison container, tell what was in it.

Directions: Answer the questions about the chart on the lines provided.

1. What is the main idea of the chart?

   The main idea of the chart is to explain how to report an emergency.

2. What kind of information is included in the third column of the chart?

   The third column tells you what to say when you call for help.

3. In which column can you find who to call in case of emergency?

   The second column tells you who to call in case of emergency.

4. What do you say when you call during a serious medical problem?

   Tell the person who answers the call where you are. Describe as much about the problem as you can.

5. What is the one thing you should say when calling for help in any emergency?

   No matter what the emergency is, tell the person on the phone where you are.

Facts on First Aid

Directions: Match the correct letter with the description.

___B___ **1.** The quick and temporary care given to a person who has a sudden illness or injury

___D___ **2.** An infection caused by poisons made by bacteria that enter a puncture wound

___A___ **3.** A method of reviving a person using mouth-to-mouth breathing and strong rhythmic pressing on the chest

___E___ **4.** Steps taken to avoid having contact with pathogens in body fluid

___C___ **5.** A break in a bone

Vocabulary
A CPR
B first aid
C fracture
D tetanus
E universal precautions

Directions: Fill in the blanks in the chart below.

First Aid for Nosebleeds and Sprains		
Injury	**Description**	**What to Do**
Nosebleed	**6.** An injury to blood __vessels__ inside the nose	• **7.** Sit down and lean __forward__. • Pinch nostrils shut for 10 minutes.
Blister	**8.** An area under the skin where __fluid__ collects.	**9.** Clean the area with __soap and water__. • Cover with a clean bandage. **10.** Don't __break__ the blister.

Facts on First Aid

Directions: Complete the lesson outline by filling in the blanks.

What Is First Aid?

1. First aid is the _____*quick*_____ and
   _____*temporary*_____ care given to a person who has
   a sudden illness or injury.

2. To treat a minor cut using first aid, follow these steps.
   a. Clean the cut with _____*soap and water*_____.
   b. Put _____*pressure*_____ on the cut.
   c. Cover the cut with a clean _____*bandage*_____.

3. To avoid having contact with pathogens in body fluid, use
   _____*universal precautions*_____.

4. Household products such as cleaners and paints can be
   _____*poisons*_____ if they are swallowed.

Rescue Breathing and CPR

5. To find if a victim is breathing, a person performing
   rescue breathing or CPR should feel for exhaled
   _____*air*_____.

6. If a person isn't breathing and doesn't have a heartbeat,
   call _____*9-1-1*_____.

7. Only people who are trained in _____*rescue breathing*_____ or
   _____*CPR*_____ should perform these actions.

8. The purpose of CPR is *to revive a person who is not breathing*
   and who has no heartbeat.

Facts on First Aid

First Aid for Minor Injuries	
Name	**First Aid Steps**
Bee sting	• Scrape the stinger out with a hard card edge or nail file. • Clean the area with soap and water. Put ice on the area. • If the person feels dizzy or can't breathe, get emergency medical care.
Blister	• Clean with soap and water. • Cover with a clean bandage. • Don't break the blister.
Nosebleed	• Sit down and lean slightly forward. Pinch your nostrils shut for 10 minutes. • Get medical help if the nose bleeds for more than 10 minutes.
Rashes from plants	• Run cold water over the area. • Use calamine lotion for itching.

Directions: Answer the questions about the chart on the lines provided.

1. What is the main idea of the chart?

   The chart gives the reader important first aid information for minor injuries.

2. What information in the chart is listed in rows?

   Each row lists a different injury and provides the first aid steps for that injury.

3. In which column are the first aid steps for a blister listed?

   the second column

4. What are the first aid steps to use for a rash from a plant?

   Run cold water over the area. Use calamine lotion for itching.

5. When should you get medical help for a nosebleed?

   if the nose bleeds for more than 10 minutes

Staying Violence Free

Directions: Match the correct letter with the description.

_____C_____ 1. Fairness for all people

_____D_____ 2. A rule that people in a community, state, or nation are required to follow

_____E_____ 3. A person who has been harmed

_____B_____ 4. Treating some people in a different way than you treat others

_____F_____ 5. A device used for violence

_____A_____ 6. Unwanted touching of a person's private body parts, for example

Vocabulary
A abuse
B discrimination
C justice
D law
E victim
F weapon

Directions: Answer the questions on the lines provided.

7. Describe one example of discrimination.

   Some possible answers: not liking someone because of his or

   her physical appearance, putting down people because of their

   race or religion

8. Name one kind of worker who helps victims of violence get justice.

   Possible answers: police; detectives, judges

9. Name a weapon used for violence against others.

   Possible answer: A gun is a weapon used for violence.

10. What is the purpose of a law?

    A law gives people in a community a rule to follow. It also helps make

    the community safer.

Name	Date

Staying Violence Free

Directions: Complete the lesson outline by filling in the blanks.

The Many Faces of Violence

1. A student who threatens to beat up another student is using a kind of violence called _____bullying_____.

2. Putting down people who have a different religion is a kind of violence called _____discrimination_____.

Dealing with Violence

3. One way to avoid violence is to manage your _____anger_____ and _____cool down_____ before you do anything.

4. One way to prevent violence is to treat others with _____respect_____ by not _____putting them down_____.

5. To avoid violence, choose friends who _____don't use violence_____ and _____get away_____ from violent situations.

6. Instead of fighting, try to resolve conflicts by _____talking_____ about disagreements.

7. If you use the Internet, tell a _____responsible adult_____ if someone tries to find out where you live.

Help for Victims of Violence

8. One important step for victims is to talk about their _____feelings_____, such as being _____afraid_____, _____depressed_____, or _____ashamed_____.

9. If one person does not believe a victim, the victim should _____find another person to talk to_____.

Resolve Conflicts

Directions: Suppose that someone drops one of your books in a puddle of water on purpose. Work with a partner to role-play ways to resolve the conflict without violence. Use the lines below to plan your role-play. The steps are listed at the right as a reminder.

1. Stay calm.
2. Talk about the conflict.
3. List possible ways to settle the conflict.
4. Agree on a way to settle the conflict. You may need to ask a responsible adult for help.

1. What will you do to stay calm?

   Students may suggest counting to 10 or taking a deep breath.

2. How will you talk about the conflict?

   Students should suggest using I-messages to make their position clear.
   They should also mention listening to the other person.

3. What ways could you settle this conflict?

   Accept reasonable answers.

4. Which choice will you use in your role-play? Will you need the help of a responsible adult to resolve this conflict?

   Answers will vary. If tempers are hot, students should suggest enlisting
   the aid of an adult to mediate.

Name

Date

Steer Clear of Gangs

Directions: Answer the following question.

1. Describe one example of what gang members might do.

   Possible answers: steal, fight, use violence, sell

   illegal drugs, kill

Vocabulary
gang

2. Write a paragraph about a student who refuses to join a gang. Include activities that the student could do instead of joining a gang.

   Students should include information on resistance skills as well as ideas

   for alternative activities to gangs.

   _____

   _____

   _____

   _____

   _____

   _____

   _____

   _____

   _____

   _____

   _____

   _____

   _____

   _____

   _____

   _____

   _____

   _____

   _____

Steer Clear of Gangs

Directions: Complete the lesson outline by filling in the blanks.

What Is a Gang?

1. A person may join a gang because he or she has _____ problems _____ at home, at school, or with friends.

2. Gang members may use hand _____ signals _____, wear specific _____ colors _____, and have _____ tattoos _____ as symbols of the gang.

3. Gang members may buy _____ illegal _____ drugs.

4. Gang members may use _____ weapons _____ to fight with or kill members of other gangs.

How to Stay Out of Gangs

5. Gang members may expect other members to behave in _____ dangerous _____ ways. Gang members could get _____ hurt _____ or even _____ killed _____.

6. If a person goes to jail for doing _____ illegal activities _____ in a gang, this can make it hard to finish _____ school _____ or get a _____ job _____.

7. Five ways you can stay out of gangs are:

   a. stay away from _____ gang members _____ and _____ places where gang members hang out _____.

   b. _____ say "no" and walk away _____ if someone pressures you.

   c. _____ spend time with your family _____.

   d. attend _____ school and school activities _____.

   e. spend time with people who _____ share your interests _____.

8. Be careful around _____ weapons _____. Never touch a _____ gun _____ you find lying around outside or in someone else's home. It might be _____ loaded _____.

Drugs and Your Health

Directions: Use the clues to complete the puzzle.

Across:

1. A(n) _____ is a strong desire to do something even though it is harmful.
2. A drug that is against the law to have, use, buy, or sell is a(n) _____ drug.
3. A medicine that can be obtained only with a doctor's written order is a(n) _____ drug.
4. Drug _____ is any use of an illegal drug or the harmful use of a legal drug.
5. A medicine that can be bought without a doctor's order is a(n) _____ drug.

Down:

6. A drug used to prevent, treat, or cure a health condition is a _____.
7. A(n) _____ is a substance that changes how the mind or body works.
8. An unwanted reaction to a drug is a(n) _____.
9. Accidental unsafe use of a medicine is drug _____.

Vocabulary
abuse
addiction
drug
illegal
medicine
misuse
over-the-counter
prescription
side effect

Drugs and Your Health

Directions: Complete the lesson outline by filling in the blanks.

Drugs Used as Medicine

1. Medicines that can be bought without a doctor's order are
   _____over-the-counter (OTC) drugs_____.

2. Medicines that can be bought only with a doctor's order
   are ___prescription drugs___.

3. A(n) _____generic_____ drug may do the same
   thing but costs less than a _____brand name_____ drug.

Safety Rules for Medicines

4. Medicines can harm you if they ___are not used safely___.

5. Seven safety guidelines for using medicines are:
   a. Take only from a responsible adult._____
   b. Follow the instructions.._____
   c. Tell the doctor and pharmacist about all medicines you take._____
   d. Take only your own medicines._____
   e. Stop taking a medicine if you have side effects._____
   f. Keep medicines in their original containers._____
   g. Check the seal on packages of OTC medicine._____

Drug Misuse and Abuse

6. The accidental unsafe use of a medicine is
   ___drug misuse___.

7. The use of a(n) _____illegal_____ drug or the
   harmful use of a legal drug is _____drug abuse_____.

8. Abusing drugs can harm both your
   _____mind_____ and your
   _____body_____.

9. Addiction can lead to ___serious health problems or death___.

Drugs and Your Health

Prescription Drug Labels

Each part of a prescription label tells important information. The abbreviation "Rx" stands for "prescription." The abbreviation "mg" stands for "milligram," a measurement of weight. To use medicine safely, read the label each time you take it. Make sure it is your medicine and follow the directions carefully.

Directions: Use information from the label. Answer the questions on the lines provided.

FAMILY PHARMACY

Rx 12543
CINDY MILLER
128 MAIN ST., NORTHTOWN, NY 12345

TAKE TWO CAPSULES
TWICE A DAY

PENICILLIN 200 MG

REFILLS: 2   Exp: 07/30/
DR. KENNETH SCOTT

1. What is the prescription number?

   Rx #12543

2. Why do you think the prescription number is important?

   Possible answer: The pharmacist uses numbers to keep
   track of all the prescriptions he or she has filled.

3. Who is the doctor who ordered the prescription?

   Dr. Kenneth Scott

4. Who is the prescription for?

   Cindy Miller

5. What is the name of the medicine? _____ penicillin _____

6. When, how often, and how much medicine is the patient supposed to take?

   2 capsules twice a day

7. What is the strength of the medicine in each capsule?

   200 mg

8. What is the expiration date? _____ 7/30 _____

9. Why is the expiration date important?

   The medicine might not be safe to use after this date.

10. How many times can this prescription be refilled?

   twice

Drugs and Your Health

Over-the-Counter (OTC) Drug Labels

To take an over-the-counter drug safely, you need to read the label every time you use it. Each part of the label tells important information. This is a sample OTC drug label.

Directions: Use information from the label. Write the answers on the lines provided.

1. What is the name of this OTC drug?

   Non-Drowsy Nasal Decongestant

2. What symptoms does this OTC drug treat?

   nasal congestion

3. What warnings does the label have, if any?

   Do not use with MAOI; do not

   use more than the recommended

   dose; stop and ask a doctor if you get nervous, dizzy or sleepless,

   or if you do not get better within 7 days

Drug Facts

Active ingredient *(in each tablet)*	Purpose
Pseudoephedrine HCl 30 mg . . . . Nasal Decongestant	

Uses temporarily relieves nasal congestion due to
■ common cold ■ hay fever ■ upper respiratory allergies

Warnings
Do not use if you are now taking a prescription monoamine oxidase inhibitor (MAOI) (certain drugs for depression, emotional conditions or Parkinson's disease) or for 2 weeks after stopping the MAOI drug. If you don't know if your prescription contains MAOI, ask your doctor or pharmacist first.

Do not use more than recommended dose.

Stop use and ask a doctor if ■ you become nervous, dizzy or sleepless ■ symptoms do not get better within 7 days

Directions
■ take the recommended dosage every 4-6 hours
■ do not exceed 4 doses in 24 hours

adults and children 12 years & over	2 tablets
children 6 to under 12 years	1 tablet
children under 6 years	ask a doctor

Expiration date: July 2015

Non-Drowsy NASAL DECONGESTANT

---

4. What is the proper dose of this drug for a person your age?

   1 tablet

5. How often is each dose to be taken?

   every 4–6 hours

6. What active ingredient(s) does this OTC drug contain?

   pseudoephedrine

7. What should be done with the drug after the expiration date?

   throw out the contents if any remain

Alcohol and Health

Directions: Write the letter of the correct answer on the line.

<u>F</u>   **1.** A person under the legal age for an action such as drinking alcohol

<u>E</u>   **2.** The state of being drunk

<u>D</u>   **3.** A drug that slows down body functions

<u>A</u>   **4.** A depressant drug found in some beverages

<u>C</u>   **5.** A measure of the amount of alcohol in a person's blood

<u>B</u>   **6.** A disease in which a person is addicted to alcohol

Vocabulary
A alcohol
B alcoholism
C blood alcohol concentration (BAC)
D depressant
E intoxication
F minor

Directions: Answer the questions on the lines provided.

7. A person drives a car even though his or her BAC is high. Why is this dangerous?

A high BAC means the person may be intoxicated. He or she can't think clearly enough or react quickly enough to drive the car safely.

8. What are the effects of intoxication?

Possible answers: harder to think clearly, poorer coordination, raised BAC

9. Why is it against the law for minors to drink alcohol?

Possible answers: to protect them from alcoholism and other diseases; to protect them from accidents

10. What diseases can alcoholism cause?

Possible answers: liver diseases such as cirrhosis and alcoholic hepatitis; heart disease; cancer; harm to the pancreas, kidneys, bones, and muscles

Alcohol and Health

Directions: Complete the lesson outline by filling in the blanks.

What Is Alcohol?

1. Alcohol slows down a person's _____brain_____
   and _____body_____.

2. People who are intoxicated are more likely to have car
   _____accidents_____.

Effects of Alcohol

3. People who have _____family members_____ with alcoholism
   or who _____start drinking_____ at a younger age have a
   greater risk of alcoholism.

4. The short-term effects of alcohol include:
   a. _____difficulty thinking clearly_____.
   b. _____poorer coordination and reaction time_____.
   c. _____stronger emotions_____.
   d. _____breaking family guidelines_____.

5. Possible long-term health effects of drinking alcohol include:
   a. _____heart_____ and _____liver_____ disease
      and _____cancer_____.
   b. birth _____defects_____.
   c. difficulty making _____responsible_____ decisions.
   d. trouble expressing emotions in _____healthful_____ ways.

Reasons Not to Drink Alcohol

6. Four reasons to say "no" to drinking alcohol are:
   a. _____any four of the ten reasons listed on page D14_____
   b. _____
   c. _____
   d. _____.

Name _____ **Date** _____

Alcohol and Health

Blood Alcohol Concentration (BAC) Chart

A BAC chart helps people understand the effects of alcohol. The chart shows how much alcohol is in a person's blood depending on how many drinks they have had. A BAC chart is based on a person's weight. This chart is for a person who weighs 150 pounds.

Directions: Answer the questions on the lines provided.

Number of drinks in one hour	0	1	2	3
BAC	0.00	0.02–0.03	0.05–0.06	0.08–0.09

1. If a 150-pound person drinks one drink in one hour, how much alcohol will be in his or her blood?

   0.02 to 0.03 _____

2. In most states, it is illegal to drive with a BAC of 0.08 and above. After how many drinks would it be illegal for the person to drive?

   two _____

3. If the person weighed less than 150 pounds, would his or her BAC after one drink be higher or lower than what's listed on the chart?

   higher _____

Name   Date

Alcohol and Health

Reasons to Avoid Alcohol

Directions: Use the chart. Answer the questions on the lines provided.

Five Reasons to Be Alcohol Free	
What You Say	**Why You Say It**
1. I want to obey laws.	It's against the law for people your age to drink alcohol. You must be at least 21 years old to buy or drink alcohol legally.
2. I want to make responsible decisions.	Alcohol can make you think less clearly. You might say or do something that you would regret later.
3. I want my senses to function at their best.	Drinking alcohol can change how your senses work. Your vision can become blurred. This makes it hard to see well and to judge distances.
4. I want to keep from having accidents.	Drinking alcohol slows down your reaction time. Suppose that you are riding your bicycle and someone steps in front of you. It would take you longer to brake or change directions if you had been drinking alcohol. You'd be more likely to hit the person.
5. I want to have healthful relationships.	Drinking alcohol changes how you respond to other people. People who depend on alcohol don't use their social skills as much.

1. What does the chart show?

   It shows five reasons to be alcohol free.

2. According to the chart, how can alcohol affect your ability to make responsible decisions?

   Alcohol can make you think less clearly. It can cause you to

   say or do things you would regret later.

3. Name a reason to be alcohol-free that is not listed on this chart.

   Answers may vary. Possible answers: I want to keep from being

   depressed; I want to stay away from fights; I want to protect myself

   from diseases; I do not want to have alcoholism.

Tobacco and Health

Directions: Use the words below to fill in the blanks.

carbon monoxide	nicotine	secondhand smoke
smokeless tobacco	tar	

1. Tobacco that is chewed or placed between the cheek and gums is called _____smokeless tobacco_____.

2. A stimulant drug found in tobacco is _____nicotine_____.

3. Exhaled smoke or smoke from the burning end of a cigarette, cigar, or pipe is called _____secondhand smoke_____.

4. A gummy substance in tobacco smoke that can kill lung cells is _____tar_____.

5. A poisonous gas found in tobacco smoke that makes it hard for blood to carry oxygen is _____carbon monoxide_____.

Directions: Answer the questions on the lines provided.

6. What does it mean to say that tobacco contains toxins?
   It means that tobacco contains poisons.

7. How do the chemicals in smokeless tobacco enter the body?
   They enter the body through the mouth or gums.

8. Why is secondhand smoke harmful?
   Possible answers: it can cause the same problems that afflict smokers, such as lung cancer and heart disease.

9. How can communities help protect people from secondhand smoke?
   Possible answer: they can make it illegal to smoke in public places such as in restaurants or on buses.

10. When carbon monoxide enters the blood, what would the heart have to do to get enough oxygen to the body?
   Possible answers: it would have to beat faster; it would have to work harder.

Tobacco and Health

Directions: Complete the lesson outline by filling in the blanks.

What Is Tobacco?

1. Tobacco is a plant that ____contains nicotine____.

2. Tobacco is illegal for ____people your age____ to use.

3. Smoked or inhaled tobacco smoke contains
   ____nicotine____, ____tar____, and
   ____carbon monoxide____.

Harmful Effects of Tobacco

4. Short-term effects of tobacco use include:
   a. ____addiction____.
   b. ____breathing problems____.
   c. ____stains and smells____.
   d. ____cost____.
   e. ____increased risk of fires and burns____.

5. Long-term effects of tobacco use include:
   a. ____heart disease____.
   b. ____lung disease____.
   c. ____stomach ulcers____.
   d. ____wrinkled skin____.
   e. ____poor teeth and gums____.
   f. ____poor senses of taste and smell____.
   g. ____pregnancy problems____.

Secondhand Smoke

6. About 3,000 nonsmokers die each year from
   ____lung cancer____ caused by ____secondhand smoke____.

7. Young people who breathe secondhand smoke are at higher
   risk for ____lung problems____.

Name   **Date**

Tobacco and Health

The graph shows the percentage of eighth graders who smoked cigarettes regularly from 1996 through 2002.

Directions: Use the graph. Answer the questions on the lines provided.

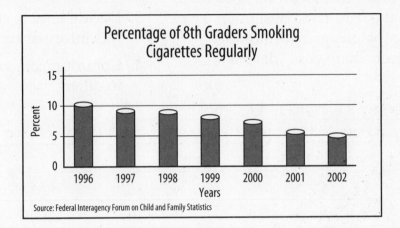

Percentage of 8th Graders Smoking
Cigarettes Regularly

Source: Federal Interagency Forum on Child and Family Statistics

1. What year does the graph begin? _____1996_____

2. What year does the graph end? _____2002_____

3. About what percent of eighth graders smoked cigarettes
   regularly in 1996? _____10_____

4. About what percent of eighth graders smoked cigarettes
   regularly in 2002? _____5_____

5. How did the percent of eighth graders who smoked
   cigarettes regularly change from year to year?
   Possible answer: It went down each year.

6. What would you predict the graph would show for 2010
   if the trend continues?
   Possible answers: less than 5%; continuing to decrease

Be a Health Advocate

Directions: Being a health advocate means giving health information to other people. The four steps for being a health advocate are listed to the right as a reminder.

With a group, brainstorm reasons not to smoke. Use the reasons to design an advertising campaign against smoking. Fill out this sheet. Share your ideas with your class.

1. Choose a healthful action to communicate.

2. Collect information about the action.

3. Decide how to communicate this information.

4. Communicate your message to others.

1. List your group's reasons not to smoke.

   Possible answers: We want healthy lungs, it costs too much, we don't

   want to smell, we don't want to get cancer.

2. What are some ways to communicate these reasons?

   Possible answers: posters, commercials, flyers, or pamphlets

3. Where will you publicize or display the information? How can you make sure that others have a chance to see, hear, read, or learn the healthful information?

   Possible answers: hang posters in hallways, play commercials over the

   intercom, hand out flyers and pamphlets

Name

Date

Other Drugs to Avoid

Directions: Write the letter of the correct answer on the line.

Vocabulary
A narcotics
B overdose
C steroids
D stimulants
E tolerance
F withdrawal

_C_ 1. Drugs that act like hormones

_F_ 2. The unpleasant reaction experienced when people who are addicted to a drug stop using it

_B_ 3. Too large an amount of a medicine or drug

_E_ 4. A condition in which more of a drug is needed in order to get the same effect

_A_ 5. Drugs that slow down the nervous system

_D_ 6. Drugs that speed up body functions

Directions: Classify each drug.

Drug	Depressant	Stimulant
7. barbiturates	X	
8. cocaine		X
9. tranquilizers	X	
10. amphetamines		X

Other Drugs to Avoid

Directions: Complete the lesson outline by filling in the blanks.

How Drug Abuse Harms Health

1. Ways in which drugs can harm health include:
   a. _addiction_____
   b. _tolerance_____
   c. _mental and physical problems_
   d. _social problems_____
   e. _legal problems_____
   f. _cost_____
   g. _withdrawal_____

Marijuana, Depressants, and Stimulants

2. Stimulants _____speed up_____ body functions, while

   depressants _____slow down_____ body functions.

3. People who abuse marijuana can have trouble

   _____learning_____ and _____remembering_____
   things.

4. Many depressants are _____legal_____ if a
   doctor prescribes them.

5. Tranquilizers and barbiturates reduce

   _____blood pressure_____ and slow

   _____the heart_____.

6. Stimulants make a person feel _____more alert_____.

7. Some people keep taking stimulants to avoid the

   _____depressed_____ feeling they get when the drug
   wears off.

8. Both legal and illegal stimulants can be

   _____addictive_____.

9. Ecstasy is an illegal drug that is both a(n)
   _____stimulant_____ and a(n) _____depressant_____.

   It can harm ____the heart and the brain____.

continued

continued

Narcotics, Inhalants, and Steroids

10. Narcotics slow down the _____nervous system_____.

11. Morphine and codeine can be prescribed by doctors for _____treating pain_____.

12. A highly addictive, illegal narcotic made from morphine is _____heroin_____.

13. An inhalant is a(n) _____chemical that is breathed_____.

14. Gasoline, paint, and some kinds of glue have harmful _____fumes_____.

15. Inhaling chemicals with harmful fumes can cause

    a. sudden _____sniffing death_____.

    b. sudden _____heart failure_____.

16. Steroids are drugs that act like _____hormones_____.

17. When used legally, steroids can:

    a. reduce _____swelling_____.

    b. help people with _____asthma or breathing problems_____.

18. Anabolic steroids are similar to a(n) _____male hormone_____.

19. Some people abuse steroids in order to _____increase their muscle size and do better in sports_____.

20. Steroids can harm the:

    a. _____liver_____,

    b. _____heart_____,

    c. _____kidneys_____, and

    d. _____reproductive_____ system.

Other Drugs to Avoid

Effects of Marijuana

Directions: The diagram shows how marijuana affects different organs and systems in the body. Use the diagram and captions to infer the answers. Write the answers on the lines.

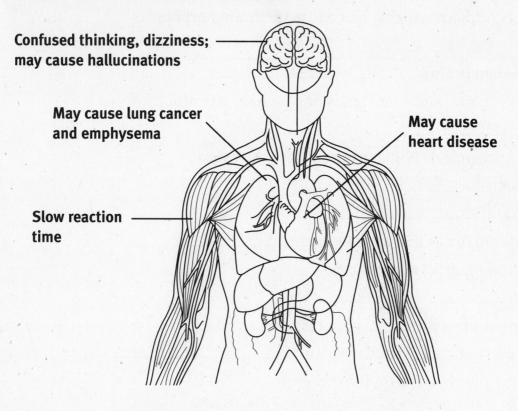

Confused thinking, dizziness; may cause hallucinations

May cause lung cancer and emphysema

May cause heart disease

Slow reaction time

1. What organs or organ systems does marijuana affect?

   brain, heart, lungs, muscles

2. Emphysema is a disease of the _____ lungs _____.

3. Marijuana can affect the brain and mind by causing

   a. hallucinations _____.

   b. confused thinking _____.

   c. dizziness _____.

4. Marijuana affects the muscles because it

   slows reaction time _____.

Other Drugs to Avoid

Effects of Inhalants

Directions: The diagram shows the effects of inhalants on the body. Use the diagram, to answer the questions on the lines provided.

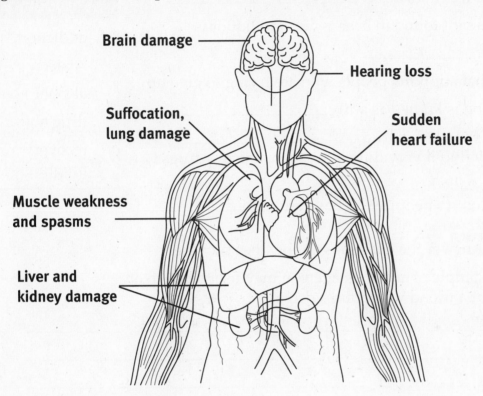

Brain damage

Hearing loss

Suffocation, lung damage

Sudden heart failure

Muscle weakness and spasms

Liver and kidney damage

1. How can inhalants affect the brain?

   They can cause brain damage.

2. What is a possible effect of inhalant abuse on the ears?

   It can result in hearing loss.

3. How can inhalants affect the lungs?

   They can cause suffocation and lung damage.

4. What can happen to the heart from abusing inhalants?

   It can suddenly fail.

5. What can happen to the arms and legs of people who abuse inhalants?

   They can suffer muscle weakness and spasms.

6. How can inhalant abuse affect the kidney and liver?

   They can be damaged.

When Someone Abuses Drugs

Directions: Fill in each blank with the term that matches the description.

1. Any use of illegal drugs is _____drug abuse_____.

2. The depressant found in beer, wine, and liquor is _____alcohol_____.

3. A group that supports people who are trying to give up an addiction is known as a(n) _____recovery program_____.

4. When a person has a drug _____addiction_____, he or she may find it very difficult to stop abusing drugs.

5. The group called _____Alateen_____ is for teens who are close to people who have addictions.

Vocabulary
addiction
Alateen
alcohol
drug abuse
recovery program

Directions: Answer the questions on the lines provided.

6. Give an example of an I-message you may use to talk to an adult about a friend who abuses drugs.

Possible answer: I feel scared when my friend abuses drugs.

_____

_____

7. Why do you think that a group which supports people who are trying to give up an addiction is known as a *recovery* program?

Possible answer: recovery means to get your health back; people in the group are trying to recover their health by overcoming addiction.

_____

8. What must a person with an addiction decide to do before entering a recovery program?

They must choose to get help; they must decide to quit.

_____

When Someone Abuses Drugs

Directions: Complete the lesson outline by filling in the blanks.

Reasons People Abuse Drugs

1. Reasons why a person chooses to abuse drugs may include one or more of these factors:
   a. family difficulties.
   b. drug abuse in the family.
   c. peer pressure.
   d. negative self-concept.
   e. depression.
   f. media influence.

Getting Help

2. If you know someone who abuses drugs, you can get help by talking to a responsible adult. The adult may know how to find help for the person. He or she can help you manage your feelings.

3. Recovery programs include:
   a. Alcoholics Anonymous.
   b. Narcotics Anonymous.

4. Family members may need help to deal with the pain and anger they feel because of the behavior of the person who abuses drugs.

Steps to Drug Recovery

Directions: Use the diagram to answer the questions.
Write the answers on the lines provided.

The diagram outlines the steps that are needed for a person
to recover from drug abuse or drug addiction. Read the steps
from bottom to top. The bottom step is the first step to drug
recovery.

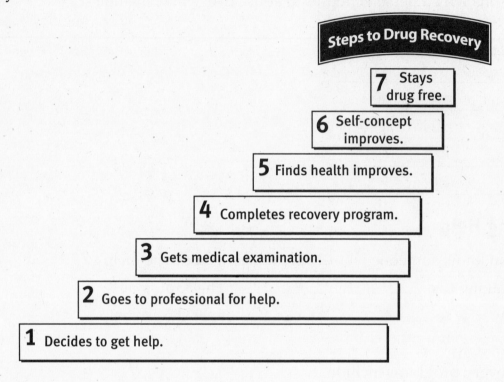

Steps to Drug Recovery

7 Stays drug free.

6 Self-concept improves.

5 Finds health improves.

4 Completes recovery program.

3 Gets medical examination.

2 Goes to professional for help.

1 Decides to get help.

1. What is the first step to drug recovery?
   The person must decide to get help.

2. What step must a person complete just before entering
   a recovery program?
   He or she must get a medical examination.

3. Besides a person's health, what else improves after recovery?
   self-concept

4. What is the final step to drug recovery?
   staying drug free

Resisting Pressure

Directions: Fill in the blanks in the puzzle. Use the terms that match the descriptions. Write each letter that has a number below it on the line with the matching number at the bottom of the page. Read the decoded message.

1. Skills that help you resist pressure to make a wrong decision

2. Choosing not to abuse drugs

3. Rules

4. A substance that changes the way the body or mind works

5. Treating others with dignity and consideration

Vocabulary
drug
regulations
resistance skills
respect
drug free

1. r e s i s t a n c e s k i l l s
                            1   2

2. d r u g   f r e e
           3   4

3. r e g u l a t i o n s
           5   6   7

4. d r u g
    8   9

5. r e s p e c t
                10

Message:

n o   d r u g   a b u s e !
1 7   8 4 3 5   6 9 2 10

Resisting Pressure

Directions: Complete the lesson outline by filling in the blanks.

Saying "No!"

1. Peers or others may _____pressure you_____ to use drugs.

2. If you are drug free, you _____choose not to abuse drugs_____.

3. When you say "no" to drug abuse, you show that you _____respect_____ yourself and are making a(n) _____responsible_____ decision.

Laws and Regulations on Drug Use

4. Some drugs that are legal for adults are _____illegal_____ for people your age.

5. You can go to jail if you _____break drug laws_____.

6. Three U.S. government departments enforce laws about drugs, tobacco, and alcohol. These are:
   a. _____Food and Drug Administration or FDA_____.
   b. _____Drug Enforcement Administration or DEA_____.
   c. _____Bureau of Alcohol, Firearms, and Tobacco, or ATF_____.

7. The FDA has regulations that tell doctors _____how to prescribe drugs safely_____.

8. The DEA enforces _____laws about illegal drugs_____.

9. The ATF deals with laws about _____alcohol_____, _____tobacco_____, and _____guns_____.

10. Besides U.S. laws, your _____state_____ and _____community_____ also have laws about drugs.

Communicable Diseases

Directions: Fill in each blank with the term that matches the description.

Vocabulary
bacteria
fungus
microbe
protozoa
virus

1. A tiny particle that makes copies of itself inside a cell is a _____virus_____.

2. A plantlike living thing made of many cells is a _____fungus_____.

3. The smallest living microbes that can reproduce on their own are _____bacteria_____.

4. Any living thing that is too small to be seen without a microscope is a _____microbe_____.

5. Simple one-celled microbes that are much larger than bacteria are _____protozoa_____.

Directions: Answer the questions on the lines provided.

6. What causes strep throat? _____bacteria_____

7. What causes flu? _____a virus_____

8. What causes athlete's foot? _____fungi_____

9. What causes malaria? _____protozoa_____

10. What type of diseases are colds, flu, and chicken pox?
_____communicable diseases_____

Name   **Date**

Communicable Diseases

Directions: Complete the lesson outline by filling in the blanks.

Types of Disease

1. Diseases that spread from person to person are
   communicable diseases.

2. _Pathogens_ cause diseases that can be spread.

3. _Noncommunicable diseases_ do not spread.

Pathogens

4. The four kinds of pathogens that cause most communicable diseases are:

   a. _viruses_   c. _fungi_

   b. _bacteria_   d. _protozoa_

5. Colds and flu are caused by _viruses_.

6. _Bacteria_ cause strep throat.

7. Ringworm is caused by _fungi_.

8. Malaria is caused by _protozoa_.

9. Pathogens are spread by _objects_,
   air, _food_,
   animals, and _water_.

How Pathogens Enter the Body

10. List five ways to reduce your risk of getting communicable diseases.

    a. _Wash your hands often_.

    b. _Don't share cups, eating utensils, or bottles_.

    c. _Keep fingers and other objects out of eyes, nose, and mouth_.

    d. _Cover your nose and mouth with a tissue when you cough or sneeze_.

    e. _Get a flu vaccine if a physician recommends it_.

How Your Body Fights Infection

Directions: Write the letter of the correct answer on the line.

_E_ 1. Cells that surround and destroy pathogens

_D_ 2. Protection from getting a particular disease

_C_ 3. A rise in body temperature

_B_ 4. Tiny hairs that line air passages

_A_ 5. A substance in blood that helps fight pathogens

Vocabulary
A antibody
B cilia
C fever
D immunization
E white blood cells

Directions: Answer the questions on the lines provided.

6. What is the stage of disease from the time a pathogen enters your body until you start showing signs of the disease?

incubation period

7. What is the stage of disease during which you show symptoms of a disease?

acute period

8. What is the stage of disease during which most symptoms go away, but you are not yet well?

recovery period

9. What happens if you relapse during the recovery period?

You go back to the acute period of the disease.

10. How does mucus protect you from pathogens?

It traps pathogens in your nose and throat.

How Your Body Fights Infection

Directions: Complete the lesson outline by filling in the blanks.

Stages of Disease

1. The three stages of disease are the ___incubation period___,
   the ___acute period___, and the ___recovery period___.

The Immune System

2. The main job of the immune system is to
   ___protect the body from disease___.

3.	First-Line Defenses
Defense	**How It Works**
skin	**a.** blocks pathogens from entering your body
b. cilia	trap pathogens in the air you inhale
c. tears	wash away dust particles and kill bacteria
stomach acids	**d.** kill many pathogens that you swallow
mucus	**e.** traps pathogens from the air

4. ___Antibodies___ fight specific pathogens.

5. Your body gets protection from a disease, or
   ___immunization___, by making ___antibodies___
   in response to a disease you had or ___to a vaccine___.

Keeping Your Immune System Strong

6. To protect your immune system, keep yourself clean,
   ___eat healthful foods___, ___drink water___, and
   ___get enough sleep___. Avoid ___smoking___
   and ___drinking alcohol___.

Name

Date

Signs of Illness

Directions: Fill in each blank with the term that matches the description.

1. A(n) _____antibiotic_____ is a drug that kills or slows the growth of bacteria.

2. _____Strep throat_____ can cause heart damage if it isn't treated.

3. Flu is caused by a(n) _____virus_____.

4. A(n) _____symptom_____ is a change in your body's condition or function that may signify disease.

Vocabulary
antibiotic
strep throat
symptom
virus

Directions: Write a paragraph that describes strep throat. Include its cause, symptoms, and how it might be treated. Be sure you use all the vocabulary words in your paragraph.

5. Students' paragraphs should include the fact that strep throat is caused by bacteria; that its symptoms include a sore throat, gray and white patches on the throat, body aches, and fever; and that a doctor may prescribe antibiotics to treat the disease.

Signs of Illness

Directions: Complete the lesson outline by filling in the blanks.

Common Signs of Illness

1. A _____symptom_____ is a change in your body's condition or _____function_____.

2. A doctor may do _____medical tests_____ to help identify a disease.

3. Two main symptoms of chicken pox are _____fever_____ and _____an itchy rash that looks like small blisters_____.

4. A "bull's-eye" rash is a symptom of _____Lyme disease_____.

Common Communicable Diseases

5. A cold is an infection of the _____respiratory system_____ caused by _____a virus_____.

6. Colds and flu can be _____treated_____ but not _____cured_____.

7. When you have a cold or flu, a doctor may tell you to _____rest_____, _____drink water_____, and take _____over-the-counter medicines_____.

8. Untreated strep throat can cause permanent _____heart damage_____.

9. A doctor may prescribe antibiotics to treat infections caused by _____bacteria_____.

10. It's important to show _____care and concern_____ for people who are ill.

Use with textbook pages D56–D59.

Name   Date

Signs of Illness

Directions: The chart lists several common communicable diseases and their symptoms. Use the chart to answer the questions.

Signs and Symptoms of Some Diseases	
Illness	**Signs and Symptoms**
Cold	Tiredness, cough, sore throat, stuffy or runny nose, sneezing, watery eyes
Flu	Fever, tiredness, cough, headache, decreased appetite, body aches, chills
Strep throat	Sore throat, gray and white patches on throat, body aches, stomach pain, fever, loss of appetite, often swelling in the throat
Chicken pox	Fever, itchy rash that looks like small blisters
Lyme disease	"Bull's-eye" rash, tiredness, headache, stiff neck, fever, chills, muscle and joint pain
West Nile virus	Fever, headaches, body aches, upset stomach. Serious cases can sometimes lead to shaking, numbness, and vision problems.

1. What information is included in this chart?

   the names of illnesses and the signs and symptoms of those illnesses

   _____

2. Where would you look to find the symptoms of a disease?

   the second column

3. What are the symptoms of strep throat?

   sore throat, gray and white patches on the throat, body aches,

   stomach pain, fever, loss of appetite, swelling in the throat

4. What does a rash in the shape of a bull's-eye tell you?

   The rash is a symptom of Lyme disease.

5. What symptoms suggest that a person has a serious case of West Nile virus?

   shaking, numbness, vision problems

Chronic Disease and the Heart

Directions: Fill in each blank with the term that matches the description.

Vocabulary
chronic disease
heart attack
heart disease
risk factor

1. A sudden loss of oxygen to the heart due to a blocked blood vessel is a _____heart attack_____.

2. A _____risk factor_____ is anything that increases the chance of loss or harm.

3. A _____chronic disease_____ lasts a long time or keeps coming back.

4. A disease of the heart or its blood vessels is _____heart disease_____.

Directions: Answer the questions on the lines provided.

5. What kind of disease is caused by heart problems present at birth?

   congenital heart disease

6. Explain what happens in coronary heart disease.

   The arteries that bring blood to the heart become narrow. This is usually
   caused by fat and cholesterol building up in the arteries.

7. How are a heart attack and a stroke similar? How are they different?

   Both can involve a blocked blood vessel. A heart attack blocks blood
   to the heart. A stroke blocks blood to the brain.

8. What is the difference between a chronic disease and an acute disease?

   A chronic disease lasts a long time or keeps coming back. An acute
   disease lasts a short time.

Name   **Date**

Chronic Disease and the Heart

Directions: Complete the lesson outline by filling in the blanks.

Chronic Disease

1. Two inherited chronic diseases are:

    a. _____cystic fibrosis_____, in which thick mucus clogs the lungs.

    b. _____sickle-cell anemia_____, in which blood cells change shape.

Heart Disease and Strokes

2. A _____stroke_____ is a sudden lack of oxygen to the brain caused by a blocked or burst blood vessel.

3. List seven warning signs of a heart attack.

    a. chest pain
    b. pain in the back, jaw, throat, or arms
    c. "heartburn" above the stomach area
    d. sweating, nausea, or vomiting
    e. difficulty breathing
    f. dizziness and fainting
    g. weakness and anxiety

Risk Factors for Heart Disease

4. Five risk factors for heart disease are

    _____heredity_____, _____high blood pressure_____,

    _____high cholesterol_____, _____smoking_____,

    and _____overweight_____.

5. Five ways to reduce your risk of heart disease are:

    a. Stay at a healthful weight.
    b. Limit the amount of fat and salt you eat.
    c. Get plenty of physical activity.
    d. Manage stress.
    e. Do not smoke.

Chronic Disease: Cancer

Directions: Write the correct letter in each blank.

1. Not normal

2. Cancerous

3. Not cancerous, or harmless

4. A disease in which cells multiply in ways that are not normal

5. A group of abnormal cells

6. A cream or lotion that protects you from the harmful rays of the sun

Vocabulary
A abnormal
B benign
C cancer
D malignant
E sunscreen
F tumor

Directions: Answer the questions on the lines provided.

7. What is the difference between a benign tumor and a malignant tumor?

A benign tumor is not cancerous and harmless. A malignant tumor is cancerous and can grow and spread.

8. What reduces your risk of getting skin cancer?

Possible answers: wearing sunscreen, avoiding the sun between 10 A.M. and 4 P.M., not using tanning lamps or booths

9. Define "cancer" in your own words. Use the word "abnormal" in your definition.

Possible answer: Cancer is a disease in which cells grow and change in abnormal ways.

10. What happens when cancer cells spread?

They destroy normal cells around them.

Chronic Disease: Cancer

Directions: Complete the lesson outline by filling in the blanks.

What Is Cancer?

1. Cancer is _____ a disease in which cells multiply _____
   _____ in ways that are not normal _____.

2. A group of abnormal cells is a _____ tumor _____.

3. A _____ benign _____ tumor is harmless.
   A _____ malignant _____ tumor is cancerous.

4. The most common types of cancer in men are
   _____ prostate _____, lung, and
   _____ colon and rectum _____ cancer.

5. The most common types of cancer in women are
   _____ breast _____, _____ lung _____,
   and colon and rectum cancer.

Preventing Cancer

6. The word CAUTION can help you remember warning
   signs for cancer. The letters in CAUTION stand for:

   a. C _____ change in bowel or bladder habits _____

   b. A _____ a sore that does not heal _____

   c. U _____ unusual bleeding or discharge _____

   d. T _____ thickening or lump in the breast or elsewhere _____

   e. I _____ indigestion or difficulty swallowing _____

   f. O _____ obvious change in a wart or mole _____

   g. N _____ nagging cough or hoarseness _____

7. If you notice any warning signs of cancer, _____ see a doctor right away _____.

8. Four healthful habits that can reduce your risk of cancer are:

   a. _____ Do not use tobacco. _____

   b. _____ Protect your skin from the sun. _____

   c. _____ Check your skin regularly for signs of skin cancer. _____

   d. _____ Eat healthfully. _____

Manage Stress

Directions: Use this sheet to practice managing stress. With a group, make a booklet for people who have ill family members. Explain how these people can use the four steps to help manage stress. Use the four steps listed in the box. Identify what advice you would include in your booklet for each step.

1. Identify the signs of stress.
2. Identify the cause of stress.
3. Do something about the cause of stress.
4. Take action to reduce the harmful effects of stress.

1. What are some common signs of stress?

   Possible answers: A person might have trouble sleeping, stomachaches or headaches, or trouble paying attention.

2. What might cause stress?

   Possible answers: A person may be worried about an ill family member. He or she may have to do more around the house to help.

3. What might people do to manage stress?

   Possible answers: Talk to a parent, guardian, teacher, doctor or friends. Show care and concern to the ill person.

4. How can people reduce the harmful effects of stress?

   Possible answer: Get physical activity to use energy and keep the body healthy so it can handle stress.

Extend

Think of another situation where these steps might be useful. On the back of this page, describe how you would use them in that situation.

Other Chronic Diseases

Directions: Fill in the grid. Use the terms that match the descriptions.

Across

1. The reaction of the body to certain substances
4. Swelling
7. A painful swelling of joints

Down

2. A chronic disease in which nerve messages in the brain are disturbed for brief periods of time
3. A chronic disease in which there is too much sugar in a person's blood
5. A chronic condition in which the small airways in the lungs become narrow
6. A device that allows a person to breathe medicine directly into the lungs

```
1a  l  l  2e  r  g  y
            p
3d          i
4i  n  f  l  a  m  m  5a  t  i  o  n
a           e           s
b           p           t
e           s           h      6i
t           y           m      n
e                   7a  r  t  h  r  i  t  i  s
s                              a
                               l
                               e
                               r
```

Directions: Answer the questions on the lines provided.

8. Explain the relationship between an allergen and an allergy.
   An allergen is the substance that causes an allergy.

9. How are a trigger and an allergen similar? How are they different?
   Both can cause reactions in the body. A trigger causes an asthma attack.
   An allergen causes an allergy.

10. What is a seizure?
    A period during which the electrical signals in the brain are disrupted

Other Chronic Diseases

Directions: Complete the lesson outline by filling in the blanks.

Diabetes

1. Diabetes is a disease in which there is too much
   _____ sugar _____ in a person's blood.

2. Type 1 diabetes usually begins in _____ childhood _____.
   Type 2 diabetes usually begins in _____ adulthood _____.

3. People with diabetes are at increased risk for blindness,
   _____ heart disease _____, and _____ kidney disease _____.

4. People who have diabetes need to check the level of
   _____ sugar _____ in their blood regularly.

5. One of the best ways to reduce your risk of type 2 diabetes
   is to _____ maintain a healthful weight _____.

Asthma and Allergies

6. In asthma, _____ small airways in the lungs _____ become narrow.

7. A person having an asthma attack may _____ wheeze _____,
   gasp for air, _____ have a dry cough _____, or feel tightness
   in the _____ chest _____.

8. In an allergy, the immune system treats an allergen like
   _____ a pathogen _____.

Epilepsy and Arthritis

9. Epilepsy is a disease in which _____ nerve messages in the brain _____
   are disturbed for brief periods of time.

10. During a seizure, the electrical signals in the brain
    _____ are disrupted _____.

11. In arthritis, joints in the body are
    _____ painfully swollen _____.

12. A person with arthritis may need _____ surgery _____
    to replace a _____ joint _____.

What Smart Consumers Know

Directions: Fill in each blank with the term that matches the description.

1. The _____media_____ are sources of news and information.

2. A(n) _____consumer_____ is a person who judges information and buys and uses products and services.

3. A(n) _____appeal_____ tries to get people to buy a product or service.

4. Something another person does that improves your health is a(n) _____health-care service_____.

5. A(n) _____generic_____ product does not have a brand name.

6. A(n) _____health-care product_____ is an item used to improve your health.

7. Companies use _____advertising_____ to sell products and services.

Vocabulary

advertising

appeal

consumer

generic

health-care product

health-care service

media

Directions: Answer the questions on the lines provided.

8. Explain how advertising and appeals are related.

   Possible answers: Advertising tries to get consumers to buy products

   and services. Appeals are statements that companies use in advertising.

9. How are healthcare products and healthcare services alike? How are they different?

   Possible answer: Both are used to improve your health. Products are

   items used by consumers. Services are things that other people do.

10. Give two examples of advertising found in the media.

   Possible answers: television commercials, radio commercials,

   advertisements printed in newspapers and magazines

What Smart Consumers Know

Directions: Complete the lesson outline by filling in the blanks.

Health-Care Products and Services

1. A ___health-care product___ is an item used for physical, mental, or social health.

2. A ___health-care service___ is something another person does that improves your physical, mental, or social health.

3. A ___consumer___ judges information and buys and uses products and services.

Choosing Wisely

4. The media include:

   a. ___TV___.

   b. ___radio___.

   c. ___magazines___.

   d. ___newspapers___.

5. Appeals are often found in ___advertisements___.

6. Before you buy a product or service, ask yourself, ___"Do I really need this?"___

Technology and Health Care

7. When you use the Internet, be sure your facts come from ___reliable___ sources. These sources include:

   a. ___the U.S. government___

   b. ___trusted health organizations___

8. It's wise to limit the TV you watch because:

   a. TV programs often show ___violence___.

   b. Watching TV takes time you might spend ___with other people___ and ___being physically active___.

   c. TV programs often show many ___advertisements___.

What Smart Consumers Know

Directions: When you are a consumer, you can get important information from product labels. This information can help you make wise choices. Use this label to answer the questions.

1. What product is this label from?

   a bottle of sunscreen

2. What is the product used for?

   to protect your skin from the sun

3. Suppose you are allergic to a chemical used in this product. Where should you look on the label?

   the list of ingredients

4. Where would you look on the label to see how strong the product is?

   the SPF number

5. What is not shown on the label that you might think about when buying this product?

   Possible answer: the price

Drug Facts	
Active ingredients	**Purpose**
Octinoxate 7.5%	Sunscreen
Octisalate 5.0%	Sunscreen
Octocrylene 9.0%	Sunscreen
Oxybenzone 6.0%	Sunscreen

Uses
- Sun Protection Factor 40 • helps prevent sunburn
- retains SPF after 80 minutes of activity in the water

Warnings
For external use only

When using this product
- keep out of eyes. Rinse with water to remove.

Stop use and ask a doctor if
- rash or irritation develops and lasts.

Keep out of reach of children. If swallowed get medical help or contact a Poison Control Center right away.

Directions
- shake well
- apply generously before sun exposure and as needed
- children under 6 months of age: ask a doctor
- reapply after towel drying, swimming or perspiring

Inactive ingredients Water, Sorbitan Isostearate, PVP/Eicosene Copolymer, Sorbitol, Stearic Acid, Triethanolamine, Aloe Barbadensis Gel, Barium Sulfate, Dimethicone, Polysorbate 20, Benzyl Alcohol, Fragrance, Methylparaben, Carbomer, Imidazolidinyl Urea, Simmondsia Chinensis (Jojoba) Seed Oil, Propylparaben, Tocopherol, Disodium EDTA.

Help for Consumers

Directions: Write the letter of the correct answer on the line.

_B_ 1. Checking the price of an item in several stores before you buy

_D_ 2. Items you spend money on

_A_ 3. A plan for spending and saving money

_F_ 4. A warning that a product is not safe

_C_ 5. People who help when there is a problem with a product or service

_E_ 6. The amount of money you expect to receive in a certain period of time

_G_ 7. A list of times, events, and things to do

Vocabulary
A budget
B comparison shopping
C consumer advocacy group
D expenses
E income
F recall
G schedule

Directions: Answer the questions on the lines provided.

8. Explain how a budget and a schedule are similar and different.

Both are tools you can use to help you plan. A budget helps you

plan how to use your money. A schedule helps you plan how to

use your time.

9. How can you use your income and expenses to plan a budget?

Possible answer: Add up all your expenses and make sure they are

less than or equal to your income.

10. How can a consumer advocacy group help you?

Possible answer: It can help me when I have a problem with a

product I bought.

Help for Consumers

Directions: Complete the lesson outline by filling in the blanks.

Protecting Consumers

1.

Government Agencies	
Agency	**What It Does**
a. Food and Drug Administration	Makes sure that food, drugs, and medical devices are safe; makes labeling rules
Federal Trade Commission	b. Makes rules about how companies can do business
Consumer Product Safety Commission	c. Warns consumers about products that are not safe; announces recalls

2. A __consumer advocacy group__ is a private group that helps consumers who have a problem with products or services.

Budgets and Schedules

3. A budget is a plan for __spending and saving money__. The four steps to making a budget are:

   a. __list your income__.   c. __plan to save money__.

   b. __list your expenses__.   d. __plan for things you want__.

4. Checking the price of an item in several stores before you buy it is called __comparison shopping__.

5. A schedule is __a list of times, events, and things to do__. Three things to do when you make a schedule are:

   a. __write down what you must do__.

   b. __add what you want to do__.

   c. __make a calendar__.

Anna's Budget

Directions: Use Anna's budget below to answer the questions.

Income	Savings	Things I Need	Things I Want
$10.00 from Aunt Julie	$3.00	New markers for art class $5.50	
$5.00 allowance		Museum ticket for field trip $5.00	

1. What is listed in the first column? _____ Income _____

2. How much income does Anna have?
   _____ $15.00 _____

3. What is listed in the third column?
   Things I Need
   _____

4. How much will Anna spend on things she needs and
   on saving? _____ $13.50 _____

5. What is the title of the fourth column?
   Things I Want
   _____

6. How much money would Anna have left to spend on
   things she wants? _____ $1.50 _____

7. Why did Anna leave the fourth column for last?
   She needs to be sure she has enough for things she needs
   and for saving before she plans to buy things she wants.
   _____
   _____

Use Communication Skills

Directions: With a partner, role-play a situation in which you might call a business about a product. Use the steps you have learned to communicate clearly. The steps are listed to the right as a reminder. The questions below can help you plan your role play.

1. Some possible situations:

   Possible answers: I have a question about

   how a product works; I want to find out the

   price of a product.

2. The situation we chose:

   Choices will vary.

3. What is the best way to communicate in this situation?

   Answers will vary but should show an understanding of different ways

   to communicate.

4. What message will the person who is calling send?

   Answers will vary but should show understanding of the situation.

5. How will we show that we are listening to each other?

   Answers should show understanding of active listening skills.

6. How will we make sure that we understand each other?

   Answers should show understanding of active listening skills.

Extend

Team up with another pair of students. Choose a situation in which more than two people need to communicate about a product or service. Role-play the situation. Try several different ways to communicate and decide which way works best. Perform your role-play for the class.

Planning a Healthful Community

Directions: Fill in the grid. Use the terms that match the descriptions.

Across:

4. _____ is doing a job without being paid.
5. Restaurant inspectors help with disease _____, to keep diseases from spreading.

Down:

1. In many communities, _____ workers remove trash.
2. Vaccines are an important part of disease _____.
3. Vaccines are also called _____.

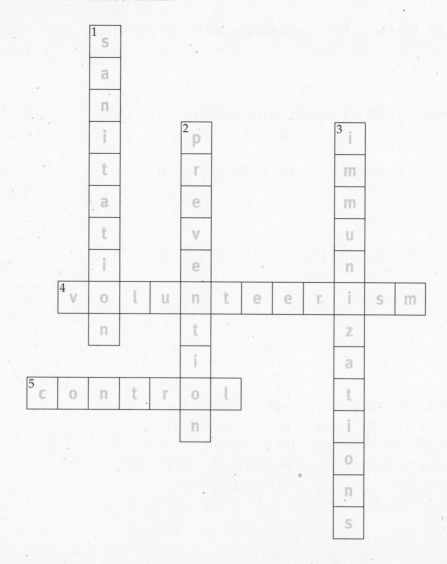

Planning a Healthful Community

Directions: Complete the lesson outline by filling in the blanks.

Community Health Needs

1. Treating water keeps people from
   getting diseases from pathogens in the water.

2. Vaccines are an important part of disease prevention.

3. Examples of disease control include:

   a. trash collection.

   b. inspecting restaurants.

Meeting Community Health Needs

4. Services that a health department provides include:

   a. teaching people how to avoid illness.

   b. offering low-cost or free vaccines.

   c. working to control diseases spread by insects.

   d. sending inspectors to make sure restaurants and markets are safe.

   e. making sure restaurant workers don't have communicable diseases.

5. The sanitation department in many communities makes sure the community is clean.

6. The water and sewer department removes
   sewage from the water.

7. The recreation department in many communities takes care of parks and playgrounds.

The Importance of Volunteers

8. Volunteers provide services without being paid.

Careers in Health and Fitness

Directions: Fill in each blank with the term that matches the description.

1. A(n) _____physical therapist_____ helps people exercise and recover after an injury or disease.

2. A(n) _____school psychologist_____ helps students solve personal problems.

3. The work that a person does throughout life is a(n) _____career_____.

4. A(n) _____school nurse_____ cares for students and teachers who become ill.

5. A responsible person who helps a younger person is a(n) _____mentor_____.

6. A(n) _____emergency medical technican (EMT)_____ gives first aid to people.

Vocabulary

career

emergency medical technician (EMT)

mentor

physical therapist

school nurse

school psychologist

Directions: Write a short description of one health career. Explain who might be a mentor for someone interested in that career.

7. Answer should show an understanding that a career is the work that a person does through life, and should choose an appropriate mentor.

_____

_____

_____

_____

_____

_____

_____

_____

_____

_____

_____

Careers in Health and Fitness

Directions: Complete the lesson outline by filling in the blanks.

Learning About Careers

1. A career is _the work a person prepares for and does throughout life_.

2. Two ways to learn about a career are:

   a. _find more information at a library_.

   b. _talk to a mentor who has the career_.

Careers in Health Care

3.

Health Careers	
Location	**Type of Career**
a. _Hospitals and doctors' offices_	Nurses, doctors, dieticians
Emergencies	b. _Emergency medical technicians_
School	c. _School nurses, school psychologists, physical education teachers, drug and alcohol counselors_
d. _Community_	Nurses, physical therapists, personal trainers

Preparing for a Career

4. When you choose a career, you should consider where you would work, _what you would do each day_, _the training you would need_, and _your interests_.

5. Four health careers are:

   a. _Possible answers:_   c. _____

   b. _Any four from page E27_   d. _____

Careers in Health and Fitness

Directions: The chart lists some careers in health care.
Use the chart to answer the questions.

Health Careers		
Career	**What They Do**	**Typical Education/Training**
Nurse Practitioner	Treat some conditions and prescribe drugs without the supervision of a doctor.	Advanced nursing courses and license. School and training last about 5–6 years after high school.
Personal Trainer	Teach people how to exercise safely. Help people meet physical fitness goals.	Certification in the type of training they do; some jobs need a college degree too. A degree takes about four years after high school.
Psychologist	Provide mental health care.	Graduate degree and license. School and training last 9–11 years after high school.

1. What information is found in each column?

   first column: name of the career; second column: what people with the

   career do; third column: what training is required

2. Which career needs the longest period of school and training?

   psychologist

3. What do psychologists do?

   provide mental health care

4. Which career needs certification and sometimes a college degree?

   personal trainer

Your Environment

Directions: Use the clues listed below to complete the crossword puzzle.

Across

4. Smog and carbon monoxide cause ____.
5. Water is an example of a ____.
6. Sunlight striking dirty air causes ____.
7. A substance that makes air, water, or land dirty is a ____.

Down

1. Substances in air, water, or land that can harm your health cause ____.
2. A loud or constant sound is ____.
3. Everything around you is your ____.

Vocabulary

air pollution
environment
natural resource
noise
pollutant
pollution
smog

Crossword puzzle solution:

1 Down: p o l l u t i o n
4 Across: a i r p o l l u t i o n
4 Down: a o n
2 Down: n o i s e
3 Down: e n v i r o n m e n t
5 Across: n a t u r a l r e s o u r c e
6 Across: s m o g
7 Across: p o l l u t a n t

Directions: Explain how the Clean Air Act has affected air pollution and smog. Explain how it has affected the amount of pollutants in the air.

8. Possible answer: The Clean Air Act has made factories and cars produce fewer pollutants. This has reduced the amount of air pollution. With less pollution in the air, less smog is made when sunlight strikes the air.

Your Environment

Directions: Complete the lesson outline by filling in the blanks.

Our Natural Resources

1. Things from nature that people need or use are
   ___natural resources___ .

2. The presence of substances in the ___environment___
   that can harm health is ___pollution___ . This can harm
   ___people___ , ___animals___ , and ___plants___
   that live there.

Air Pollution

3. Three major air pollutants are:

   a. a gas produced by cars, trucks, and buses called
   ___carbon monoxide___ .

   b. a gas produced by power plants that burn coal and oil,
   called ___sulfur dioxide___ .

   c. a haze from sunlight striking polluted air, called
   ___smog___ .

4. Two major causes of indoor air pollution are:
   a. ___secondhand smoke___ .   **b.** ___radon___ .

5. Loud or constant sound is ___noise___ . It
   can damage cells in the ___ear___ and
   cause ___hearing loss___ and ___stress___ .

Cleaning Up the Air

6. Five things you can do to reduce air pollution are:
   a. ___use electricity sparingly___ .
   b. ___walk or ride your bike when possible___ .
   c. ___do not smoke___ .
   d. ___plant trees___ .
   e. ___do not burn trash___ .

Set Health Goals

Directions: Think of an action you could take to reduce pollution. Use the steps for setting goals to help you make a plan to take the action. The steps are listed at the right to remind you. Write a Health Behavior Contract for your plan. Use the back of this page to write your contract.

1. Write the health goal you want to set.

2. Explain how your goal might affect your health.

3. Describe a plan you will follow to reach your goal. Keep track of your progress.

4. Evaluate how your plan worked.

1. The action I would take:

   Possible answer: Plan to ride my bike to my friends' homes instead of asking for a ride.

2. How this action might affect my health:

   Answers should reflect an understanding of the goal and how it will reduce pollution.

   Possible answer: I would get more exercise and reduce air pollution.

3. My plan and how I will keep track:

   Answer should include a clear plan and a way to keep track of progress.

   Possible answer: I will keep track of the times I ride my bicycle on a chart.

4. How I will evaluate my plan:

   Answers should include a way to revise the plan if it does not succeed. Possible answer: I will look at my chart after a week. I will ask my parents to remind me.

Extend

Set a class goal to do something to reduce pollution. With your teacher's permission, choose an action that you can do as a class. Plan what you will do. Follow your plan. Evaluate how your action will help your health and your community's health.

Protecting Water and Land

Directions: Fill in each blank with the term that matches the description.

1. A(n) _____open dump_____ is an area where waste is left on the ground.

2. A(n) _____incinerator_____ burns trash and other waste.

3. Trash is buried in a(n) _____landfill_____ and covered with soil and clay.

4. Waste that contains substances that are harmful to people is _____hazardous waste_____.

5. Harmful substances in a river, lake, or ocean cause _____water pollution_____.

6. Harmful substances on or in the soil cause _____land pollution_____.

7. A _____sanitary landfill_____ has a plastic or clay liner to keep wastes from leaking into soil, lakes or rivers.

8. Trash that people drop on the ground is called _____litter_____.

Vocabulary
hazardous waste
incinerator
land pollution
landfill
litter
open dump
sanitary landfill
water pollution

Directions: Answer the questions on the lines provided.

9. Explain why sanitary landfills make less land pollution than open dumps.

Possible answer: Open dumps are uncovered and allow waste to leak into soil. Sanitary landfills are covered and have liners, so wastes do not leak into the soil.

10. Explain how using an incinerator can reduce pollution.

Possible answer: Trash is burned in the incinerator, so it won't pollute soil or water. Filters on the incinerator reduce air pollution.

Protecting Water and Land

Directions: Complete the lesson outline by filling in the blanks.

Water Pollution

1. Three sources of water pollution are:

   a. chemicals used to kill weeds and insects _____.

   b. chemicals and wastes from factories _____.

   c. sewage _____.

Land Pollution

2. Litter is _____ trash that people drop onto the ground _____.
   It causes problems because it:

   a. makes an area look dirty _____.

   b. attracts rodents and insects that carry pathogens _____.

   c. can wash into rivers and oceans when it rains _____.

3. Areas where waste is dumped and left on the ground are ___ open dumps ___.
   Waste from them can attract ___ pests ___ and ___ seep into ___ soil.

4. Substances that are harmful to people or animals
   cause ___ hazardous waste ___.

Reducing Water and Land Pollution

5. Two laws that have reduced water pollution are the
   ___ Clean Water Act ___ and the ___ Safe Drinking Water Act ___.

6. Three ways you can reduce water pollution are:

   a. dispose of chemicals properly _____.

   b. dispose of trash properly _____.

   c. volunteer to help clean up rivers, lakes, or other bodies of water _____.

7. Communities have replaced open dumps with
   ___ sanitary landfills ___ and ___ incinerators ___.

8. Three ways you can reduce land pollution are:

   a. don't throw litter on the ground _____.

   b. pick up trash _____.

   c. recycle paper, cans, and glass and plastic containers _____.

Conservation

Directions: Write the letter of the correct answer on the line.

__B__ 1. Coal, oil, and natural gas burned to get energy

__D__ 2. A resource that can be replaced within a normal lifetime

__C__ 3. A resource that can't be replaced within a reasonable amount of time

__A__ 4. The protection and careful use of natural resources

Vocabulary
A conservation
B fossil fuels
C nonrenewable resource
D renewable resource

Directions: Answer the questions on the lines provided.

5. Give three examples of power that is generated using renewable resources.

Hydropower, solar power, and wind power

6. Are fossil fuels renewable or nonrenewable resources? Explain your answer.

Nonrenewable; they cannot be replaced within a normal lifetime.

7. Why is taking shorter showers an example of conservation?

Possible answer: You can save as much as 20 gallons of water, which

is a resource that people need.

8. What is energy?

The ability to do work. It also refers to fuels used for heat and

electricity and to run cars and trucks.

9. Give two examples of energy conservation.

Possible answers: turning off lights, turning down the heat

10. Explain how conserving energy conserves natural resources.

Possible answer: Most energy is created using fossil fuels, which

are nonrenewable resources. If we conserve energy, we also

conserve those resources.

Conservation

Directions: Complete the lesson outline by filling in the blanks.

Conserving Water Resources

1. Conservation is the ___protection___ and ___careful use___ of natural resources. It is important because many resources are___limited___.

2. Five ways to conserve water are:
   a. ___take short showers instead of baths___.
   b. ___run only full loads in washing machines and dishwashers___.
   c. ___don't run the water while brushing teeth or washing your hands or face___.
   d. ___throw tissues and other waste in the trash instead of in the toilet___.
   e. ___tell an adult about leaky pipes or faucets___.

Conserving Energy

3. Energy is ___the ability to do work___. Most energy today comes from ___nonrenewable___ resources. These resources ___cannot be replaced___ within a reasonable amount of time.

4. Three fossil fuels are:
   a. ___coal___. b. ___oil___. c. ___natural gas___.

5. Three renewable energy sources are:
   a. ___solar power___. b. ___wind power___. c. ___hydropower___.

6. Renewable energy sources will not ___run out___.

7. Six ways to conserve energy are:
   a. ___use natural light instead of a lamp___.
   b. ___turn off lights when you leave a room___.
   c. ___use compact fluorescent bulbs___.
   d. ___put on a sweater instead of turning up the heat___.
   e. ___use a fan instead of an air conditioner to keep cool___.
   f. ___dry clothes on a clothesline___.

Conservation

Directions: Use the graph below to answer the questions.

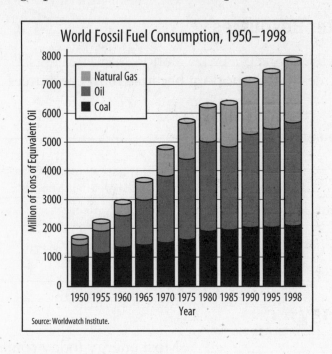

World Fossil Fuel Consumption, 1950–1998

Million of Tons of Equivalent Oil

Natural Gas
Oil
Coal

1950 1955 1960 1965 1970 1975 1980 1985 1990 1995 1998
Year

Source: Worldwatch Institute.

1. What does this graph show?

   the amount of fossil fuels used in the world

2. What time span does the graph show?

   1950–1998

3. What fuel provided the smallest share of the energy used in 1980?

   natural gas

4. The use of which fuel has changed least in the years shown
   on the graph?

   coal

5. Overall, has the total use of fossil fuels increased or
   decreased in the time shown on the graph?

   increased

6. Describe how the use of the three fossil fuels has changed
   in the time shown on the graph.

   Possible answer: The fraction of energy produced by natural gas

   has increased most over the years, while the fraction produced by

   coal has decreased most.

A Positive Environment

Directions: Fill in each blank with the term that matches the description.

1. When you reduce waste, you _____precycle_____.

2. When you _____reuse_____ something, you use it again instead of throwing it away.

3. The _____visual environment_____ is everything a person sees.

4. A _____positive environment_____ promotes all kinds of health.

5. To _____recycle_____ is to change waste products so they can be used again.

Vocabulary
positive environment
precycle
recycle
reuse
visual environment

Directions: Explain how precycling, reusing, and recycling help the environment.

6. Answer should show an understanding that precycling, reusing, and recycling reduce waste and keep the environment cleaner and healthier.

Name

Date

A Positive Environment

Directions: Complete the lesson outline by filling in the blanks.

Precycle, Reuse, and Recycle

1. Precycling, reusing, and recycling materials help resources __last longer__.

2. To precycle is to __take actions to reduce waste__. To do this, choose items with __less packaging__.

3. When you reuse something, you __use it again__ instead of __throwing it away and buying a new one__.

4. To recycle something is to __change it__ so it can be __used again__.

A Positive Environment

5. A positive environment promotes __physical__, __mental and emotional__, and __family and social__ health.

6. In a positive environment:
   a. you feel __safe__ and __good about yourself__.
   b. you know that people around you __support you__ and __care about you__.
   c. your friends, family, and other people __encourage you to do your best__.

7. Four ways you can help make your environment positive are:
   a. __compliment other people when they do something positive__.
   b. __avoid saying negative things about others__.
   c. __make your home environment positive__.
   d. __help make the visual environment positive__.

8. When your __visual environment__ is attractive, you feel better about __where you live__.